Mastering Body Mechanics

A Visual Guide For Bodyworkers Incorporating the Mind-Body Connection

by Marty Morales, Certified Rolfer™

To my wife, Elena, for her neverending love and support.
To my mom, my grandmother, and my brother, who set me on the right path.
To my teachers and my students, who continue to make me grow and learn.

ACKNOWLEDGEMENTS

Thank you to Art Riggs, my friend and mentor, for his generosity and support in my career. If any of these photos display great body mechanics, it is because of his amazing training.

To Eve Gutierrez, Denise DeShetler, and Jamie Leigh Chan, thank you for being willing to get on my table and be my "super" models. I have learned from you greatly.

To PF Dumanis, thank you for your fantastic design and work in putting this book together. I appreciate all the feedback and amazing insight.

To Laura Dean, thanks for your illustration contribution and your insightful feedback.

MASTERING BODY MECHANICS

INTRODUCTION

Why do we strain? Why do we 'muscle' it? 'Muscling' refers to the unnecessary use of muscular action. Throughout our lives there are many instances where 'muscling it' has been completely unnecessary, but nevertheless a fascinating phenomenon. When we are riding a roller coaster we hold on to the safety bar or the handlebar even though we are securely strapped in or if we are in the safety of a movie theater but watching a thrilling or suspenseful movie, we find ourselves gripping the armchair or the person along side us for dear life. I propose that these reactions to everyday normal occurrences and most causes of improper body mechanics come from the same root.

What is the next step in our evolution as bodyworkers? This is a question I have been asking myself for the past eight years. In doing bodywork, I have found that we still have a lot to learn when it comes to how we use our bodies. With every year we collectively evolve and improve as bodyworkers. This evolution can have a profound and positive influence on the way we use our bodies, or Body Mechanics. This evolution in skillset unfortunately has not equated into better body mechanics. There is a stronger force that has an impact on body

mechanics than the improvement of skillsets. This has led me to discover that improper body mechanics are due in a large part to a stress response related to the 'muscling' actions previously described. To answer my initial question, the next step in our evolution as bodyworkers is to pursue mastery in body mechanics.

Back in massage school during our practicum time I was doing work on a fellow classmate and performing an effleurage on his hamstrings. "You need to go harder, I'm not feeling anything at all" he said. Not knowing anything other than the effleurage, petrissage, and maybe some tapoutement if I was lucky, I proceeded to perform a harder version of the effleurage, with more downward pressure. I felt the pressure of wanting to do a good job. I felt that if I couldn't do what my classmate asked of me, how could I turn this new vocation into a career? So, not knowing anything other than what my life had shown me up to those 32 years, I powered my way through the strokes, using my muscle to perform a stroke that was intended to be more of a flowing, relaxing stroke, the effleurage stroke, up his hamstrings. Twenty minutes and many beads of sweat later, my classmate

2

was happy, telling me he liked the pressure. Unfortunately, my wrists were hurting as a result and I had the bad feeling that I couldn't pursue this career if this was how every session was going to be like.

Seven years earlier, I had acquired the symptoms of carpal tunnel syndrome and those same feelings were making themselves evident in my right hand. My carpal tunnel symptoms had my right hand incapacitated to the point where I was wearing a wrist brace, taking anti-inflammation medication, and I was looking down the barrel of inevitable surgery. Fortunately, with some dietary changes, trigger point therapy, acupressure, and strength training, I had my wrist and my life back in just four weeks.

It was now seven years later and I was in massage school. I had the definite sense of terror as I thought, "I can't do this type of work, my wrist is killing me, I should just quit now." The instructor during that class passed by a few times but I didn't get any instruction or correction of my body mechanics. It wasn't until I got into a deep tissue class that I realized I was unnecessarily straining myself and using

the wrong tool for the job! If I could go back in time and be witness to myself doing that practicum, I would have offered myself and the classmate some advice on body mechanics, straining yourself, and avoiding injury. To this day this event several years ago sticks with me as an example of not using the right tool for the job but also for the huge need of understanding and educating massage therapists on proper body mechanics.

Since then I have explored this thing we call body mechanics, have asked myself the questions I posed earlier, and I have come up with a few proposals for answers. These thoughts have been derived into principles which have helped me throughout my career and have helped countless of my students. This book is a snapshot in time of my current findings in body mechanics. We are always growing as practitioners and this book will also add to your body of work as the information in it has helped me develop into a better bodyworker. As you can tell by now, this book is more than just a 'how-to' but also a 'how come'. If we explore the 'how-come', the 'how-to' will develop quicker, with little outside directing, and with more permanency in ourselves.

MASTERING BODY MECHANICS

CHAPTER 1:

GETTING TO WRITE THIS BOOK

My teaching of body mechanics has come out of observing my students, learning from them and from my own contemplations of the matter. Clients have also been my teachers. I have told many students a quote I was told (the source escapes me so forgive the unintentional plagiarism) "Some of the best teachers you will ever have will be the ones that show up on your table". These teachers have helped me find different ways of working and different ways of using my body. In turn, I share with my students my findings and they teach me as I see them embody these findings and figure them out in their body.

I find it a testament to proper body mechanics that I am now a Certified Rolfer™ and bodywork educator. Being in this position, I have been able to see both sides of the body mechanics dilemma. I have seen how one as a bodyworker can fall into the trap of filling up your work plate to the point where body mechanics suffer and injury results. I have seen students acquire bad habits early on that only come to rear their ugly head in the future.

There is no one rule of law that will apply for everyone as far as body mechanics is concerned. We all have different bodies and different limitations with our bodies. If anybody comes to you with an attitude of "behold my Body Mechanics glory! This is the one and the only way" quietly slip out of the classroom!

What I intend to do in this book is the following:

1. To explain why we strain, 'muscle it' and employ improper body mechanics via a physiological, psychological, and cultural approach.

2. To show a way of achieving proper body mechanics by first implementing a grounding practice

3. To show effective and no-strain ways of using your body that will help for both Western Massage Therapy (Swedish) and for Deep Tissue Massage.

In order to fulfill the above goals, we need to understand a bit about our culture, physiology and psychology and we need to gain an understanding of our bodies that we may not have had before. When I teach body mechanics, I not only help the student explore the physical aspects of employing proper body use, but I start my teachings by exploring the mind.

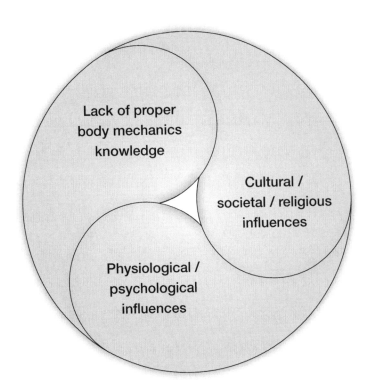

The three main reasons for improper body mechanics

I believe improper body mechanics are due in part for three main reasons:

1. Cultural/Societal influences

2. Physiological/Psychological

3. Lack of knowledge of proper body mechanics

Any decent attempt to contemplate body mechanics begins with exploring how come we do the things we do. As I asked before, why do we strain when we actually don't need to? A more precise question could be: Why do we strain and employ improper body mechanics when we might already know proper body mechanics? There is an internal innate program in our bodies that is manipulated by internal and external forces. This program is inherent in our nervous system and the external forces can be called society, culture, or just plain life as we currently know it. The internal forces can be called perception and emotions.

In our pursuit of mastery of body mechanics, we can derive principles that we can employ not only for doing bodywork, but to create a healthier living philosophy for our everyday life.

I have asked students directly what they believe is their reason for 'muscling' it and they have described to me that getting stressed out over wanting to do things right or doing a good job is the primary reason.

The above three reasons for improper body mechanics are all interrelated. One affects the others and one is affected by the others. Cultural/societal influences can affect the lack or the amount of proper body mechanics knowledge or even the desire to learn proper body mechanics. Society also influences our physiological and psychological reactions and those in turn affect proper body mechanics. Our own perceptions of what proper bodywork should feel like also affects our body mechanics.

The Best Way to Use This Book

Employing proper body mechanics in your practice is a thing that is alive and dynamic. Doing so involves going through the motions, experiencing it in your body, and examining for yourself the possibilities and the movements you are capable of. Simply reading this book and assuming you can master body mechanics can be the same as reading a book on modern dance or judo and assuming you can perform either one with proficiency. My recommendation is to read this book and to workshop the subject matter. Gather in groups of three and when you are working, designate roles: Practitioner, Observer, and Recipient. Rotate roles so everyone gets a chance to observe, to practice, and to receive bodywork using proper body mechanics. This is the best way to embody the work. Note the word 'embody' means to bring into your body.

The photos in this book are a snapshot in time and although they reflect the way I work, are still static and do not reflect the movements that may be going on. For this reason it is even more important to use the photos as a guide and attempt them in your triad workshop. Remember to not attempt to completely mimic the photos. Your body is different, unique and will tell you the best way to utilize it if you listen.

CHAPTER 2:

HOW COME?

AN EXPLORATION OF THE THREE ASPECTS OF IMPROPER BODY MECHANICS

CULTURE / SOCIETY

> *"You've got to work hard,*
> *You've got to work hard,*
> *If you want anything at all."*
>
> — *Depeche Mode, "Work Hard"*

"Work hard!!!"

We live in a society that is filled with opportunity for the enterprising individual. Most of us believe that with hard work, we can achieve anything. Unfortunately, it is the act of adhering to that concept that can hold us back. The concept of 'hard' can put us at a disadvantage when it comes to almost any aspect of our lives.

We as a culture and a society (and I'm including almost every society out there) have come to admire the term 'hard' as it relates to our work and our efforts.

When JFK made his famous Space Race speech, he said, "We choose to go to the moon...and do the other thing not because they are easy, but because they are hard." People cheered and applauded in approval. Essentially, everyone cheered for 'hard work!' JFK (brilliantly I might add) did not say "...because it's smart." No, the everyday 'Joe' wouldn't understand that. He knew the masses understand 'hard work' as something to be admired.

The mentality still stands today. When a reporter asked a certain 2008 former vice-presidential candidate's spokesperson how the candidate was able to finish an autobiography in such a short span of time, the spokesperson answered, "She worked really hard." I wonder if that entailed hitting the keyboard especially hard to get the book out sooner.

This mentality might have stemmed from our agriculture days and fed into our industrial revolution years. We might have believed that since tilling the soil and farming the land is a lot of work, that it should be hard, that it should hurt and that we should 'break our backs' doing it. Manual labor is associated with 'hard work'. What if we looked at manual labor not as hard but as 'a lot of work' or 'difficult work' or even more precisely what it is, 'physically demanding work,' one that actually requires us to use proper body mechanics in order to decrease the risk of injury? We would then change our understanding of what 'working hard' really means and do away with the term before it irrevocably embeds itself into our perception of bodywork.

We are Pre-programmed to Accept Hard Work

As I've told my students in the past, we as a society look up to and revere the term, 'HARD.' We are motivated by this term and we learn to love and receive love when we do things this way. When you didn't do well on a test in school, what did your parents tell you? They told you to 'study harder.' We strive to impress our parents and our peers and so we end up 'studying harder,' without really knowing what it means. We have progressed so much in the way we learn and teach and think and yet we are still hearing the term "study harder!" Nobody ever told me to study 'smarter.'

It's no wonder that since we spend all our lives doing things this way ('hard'), that we go into massage thinking it needs to be done 'hard' in order to be done well. This is what I thought when my classmate of long ago told me he wanted more pressure on his hamstrings. This is one of the most difficult things to deal with as a student of this practice.

At work we reward the 'hard worker'. You hear it from managers, and colleagues and we take it as a good thing to be called a 'hard worker.'

Before I was a bodyworker I was a corporate finance guy, working in finance and accounting for some good size corporations. Over and over again I would hear 'he's a hard worker' or 'thank you for all your hard work'. It goes on and on. I also remember coming home to a deliciously home-cooked meal and being told, "I know you've worked hard today". Fortunately, I haven't worked hard in years and the delicious home cooked meals haven't stopped! It was only until I started taking massage classes that I learned I didn't need to work hard in order to be effective. I realized I could work 'smart' and do an even better job. Unfortunately, we still value 'hard work' for some reason assuming that the sweat from the brow will or might always bring success. I wish we could take this word out of our vocabulary for a bit and bring in something else in its place. Working 'hard' doesn't make sense.

Working with and on people can take a toll on your daily energy but it is no excuse for the amounts of injuries that massage therapists/bodyworkers are acquiring. Back in 1992 Maja Evans wrote in her book, "The Ultimate Hand Book" that 80% of the massage therapists in practice fall out of practice within the first couple of years due to injury. This statistic has not changed dramatically in the last ten years. Have we as a group come to accept injury and the short career span of a bodyworker as a given? What if this wasn't the case? What if we could do this work well into our 90's? Proper body mechanics plays a key role in injury prevention.

Understanding that this cultural perception has reached its tendrils into our psyche uncovers an issue: A massage student goes through life not only accepting but admiring all things 'hard' and then he/she might go into a massage/bodywork class of mine and be told to not work hard. It's an extreme thought to have! It's in our culture, our language, it means something to us to 'work hard'...and in most cases, something positive and something to be admired.

It is because of this pre-programmed thought process that most massage students/therapists find themselves experiencing injuries and body issues. And here's another aspect: If massage therapists/bodyworkers experience this, shouldn't it be the case that our clients also fall into this mentality and also fall under the habit of working 'hard' and in most cases, working too 'hard'…to the point that they too will succumb to injury? As with bodyworkers, if our client wants to acquire a healthier habit, then a venture into the mind will also be necessary.

Not only do we need to unlearn this 'hard' mentality, but we also need to acquire another option for working and be able to acknowledge that we can span between options.

This is key so I will repeat it: Understanding that working 'hard' or doing 'hard massage' will not serve the bodyworker is essential for a successful practice. The other piece is understanding that banishing that mentality will be extremely difficult if not, impossible. Instead, it is key to understanding that one as a bodyworker can span this spectrum: You can work 'hard' when (or if) you need to and you can work 'smart' when it serves you and the client better.

Physiological / Psychological

*"Work it, make it, do it, makes us
Harder, better, faster, stronger…."*

**— Daft Punk,
"Harder Better Faster Stronger"**

Knowing that the term 'hard' exists or that it pervades and permeates our psyche and thus affects the way we use our bodies (especially in massage/bodywork) is not enough to get us to a point of understanding proper body mechanics. In order to reach the next level of understanding, we also need to understand what happens in our brain/mind and in our bodies that takes us down the path of 'hard' massage/bodywork.

We as bodyworkers have put ourselves in an interesting situation. We want to do a good job, for our clients and for ourselves. This desire to do well can put an inordinate amount of pressure on us. This pressure imposed or self-imposed is a form of stress. For example, we might feel stressed to 'fix' someone's injury in a short amount of time or to get tissue tightness that has accumulated over years to drastically diminish in just an hour session.

Stress can occur on many levels. Stress could have been what brought us down from the trees or pushed us to start using tools.

In any case, stress can bring about the biological phenomenon called "Fight or Flight" (FOF).

This response, 'fight or flight', was first described by Dr. Walter Cannon at Harvard University during the late 1920's.

Before we go into FOF, let's first briefly discuss the Human Nervous System (see Figure 1).

This breakdown is oversimplified and the actual interactions are much more complex. The Human Nervous system is divided into the Central Nervous System and the Peripheral Nervous System. The Central Nervous System is made up of the Brain and Spinal Cord. The Peripheral Nervous System is made up of the Autonomic and Somatic Nervous Systems. The Somatic Nervous System deals with voluntary movement of the body. The Autonomic Nervous System (ANS) deals with systems that we usually aren't conscious of (heart rate, digestion, etc.). The ANS is broken down even further into the Parasympathetic (PNS) and Sympathetic (SNS) Nervous Systems. The PNS deals with 'resting state' activities, such as digestion. The SNS is what we are most interested here both as this response can dominate our basic elements of touch and as we try to calm this response in our clients. The SNS deals with our body's response under stress and creating our "Fight or Flight" response.

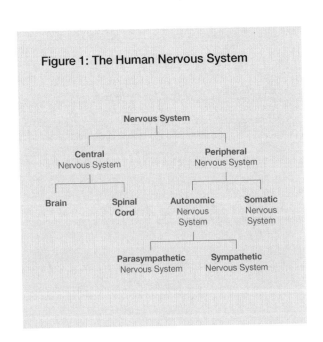

Figure 1: The Human Nervous System

Figure 2: A Representation of the Parasympathetic and Sympathetic Nervous Systems

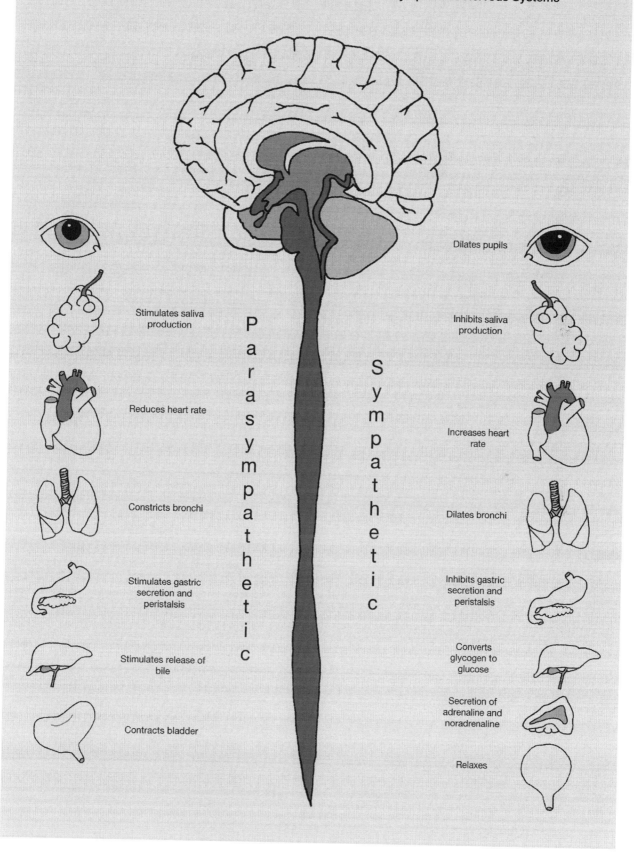

During the physiological reaction of "fight or flight," our bodies will react to stress in a unique manner. Our sympathetic nervous system will be stimulated due to stressors and we will either ready ourselves to fight or to flee; in ancient times we could have fled from the predator or we could have prepared to fight against an aggressor. Because we are readying for some sort of action, the fight or flight response entails the transfer of blood from our core to our appendages. The following is a list of actions that occur during FOF:

1. Preparation for muscular action or increase in muscular effort

2. Increase or speeding up of reflexes

3. Slowing down or stopping of digestion

4. Pupil Dilation

5. Shaking or trembling

6. Decreasing peripheral vision

The transfer of blood from our core to our appendages is what interests us here when exploring its relations to improper body mechanics. This transfer of blood causes blood to leave our torso/core/bellies and to go to our arms and legs, where we would presumably need it for muscular action. The blood is transferred out since the body believes the arms and legs will be used in order to fight or to flee. Note that blood vessels to larger muscles are dilated, however blood supply to non-vital muscle tissue is constricted which is why a person may experience cold hands and/or feet during a FOF response.

Imagery Exercise

Imagine your first experience at the dentist's office. You weren't sure what was going to happen but you had heard from your friends or family members about what to expect. Maybe they tried to reassure you that the visit would be pleasant yet you were still a bit nervous. At the dentist everyone is friendly (hopefully) but then you are seated in this strange chair with bright lights on you and a tray of metal instruments near your head. All of them ready to be used in your mouth. At some point you notice that you are gripping the chair arms with a grip of death. Even though you want to be 'grown up' and not show anyone you're afraid, you cannot hide the fact that your body is reacting in a certain way by tensing up and grasping at the chair. In effect, you are having a FOF response to being at the dentist! If you still get nervous at the dentist or maybe during a job interview, notice what happens in your body. Do your hands get cold? Do you find yourself tensing up your muscles? Do your toes curls up? I have seen these and many other reactions in a nervous massage therapist!

In modern day, we don't have the types of emergencies we had in prehistoric times but we do have modern day 'stresses'. A job deadline, a traffic ticket, or even a schedule full of back to back clients can cause a stress response in us. It's important to note that even a positive event can create a stress response. Hans Selye, who coined the term 'stress' wrote in his book, "The Stress of Life" that there are two different types of stress, 'distress' and 'eustress' where the latter is stress related to a positive event (receiving a promotion, going up to accept an award, etc.).

It has been noted that our bodies will go into a form of FOF response when we are put in stressful situations. Most of us may not go into full FOF but our bodies will exhibit some of the reactions to a FOF situation.

A classic textbook example of the flight or fight stress response depicts a zebra calmly grazing on grass. When he spots a lion closing in for the attack the stress response is activated and it applies intense muscular efforts to run away and escape. Modern medicine has determined that even though we are no longer in danger of being attacked by a lion or tiger, our urban existence has created other forms of stress and unfortunately these forms are chronic, in other words, sustained and longer lasting. The chronic stress of traffic while we are late for work, getting chewed out by the boss, the customer complaint, the murder count on the nightly news, are all types of stress we did not have before and they are affecting our bodies in ways we had not experienced before. According to the 2001 poll, "Attitudes in the American Workplace VII" which consisted of a telephone poll by Harris Interactive, it was reported, "Stress: More than a third of workers (35%) say their jobs are harming their physical or emotional health and 42% say job pressures are interfering with their personal relationships; half say they have a more demanding workload this year than last."

It has been noted, recorded and research that prolonged stress responses results in a chronic suppression of the immune system. Have you seen a massage therapist colleague with a repetitive strain injury go from bad to worse extremely quick? Although we know that every individual is different and their reactions to injuries vary greatly, this is a curious phenomenon that I've witnessed often. A self employed massage therapist knows that if he or she can't work, then they don't get paid. This makes having an injury very stressful since not being able to work for several weeks while an injury heals can drastically affect the bottom line. The question from witnessing this phenomenon is: Could the stress of having an injury make the stress response greater and lead to more 'muscling', more improper body mechanics and therefore lead the bodyworker even further down the path of injury and dis-ability? Are we stressing out over stressing out?

FACT:

Only 15% of our total cardiac output goes to muscles during a state of rest, but during strenuous activity (such as exercise or activity during Fight or Flight) about 60% to 70% of our cardiac output goes to muscles.

As we now know, a stress response doesn't necessarily need to come from a life threatening predator but can be part of our everyday 'stressors'. These everyday stressors, if occurring on a constant basis, can create a chronic cycle of stress. Normal everyday stressors can include:

1. Traffic

2. Fight with a spouse/boss/friend

3. Problems at work/school

4. Leaky faucet

For a bodyworker, stressors can include:

1. A full day of back to back massages

2. A client that requests something you may not be able to provide (such as 'hard' massage)

3. A difficult client

4. And the biggest stressor of them all: "Wanting to do a good job"

I've taught various body mechanics classes with beginning students and with experienced massage therapists. When I ask them, "What do you think the big stressor is for you that may make you strain and start to muscle it", they overwhelmingly respond, "Wanting to do a good job". This is common for bodyworkers. Most if not all bodyworkers enter into this profession because they want to help people. It is this wanting to help people that can become self-imposed pressure and thus muscle exertion

and 'muscling'. Eventually, we find ourselves down the road to improper body mechanics because of this pressure and eventual 'muscling'. This is a clear connection between the cultural/societal (perceiving 'hard work as something to be admired), the psychological (the self-imposed pressure to do a good job and work hard doing it) and the physiological (stressing out over wanting to do a good job and make others happy and then entering into a FOF response over it) as one feeds the other to create an end product of improper body mechanics and possible injury.

Understanding all these aspects of improper body mechanics I ask the following questions:

1. Could a bodyworker that has a schedule full of clients or has imposed upon him/herself the pressure to do a good job to impress their client or to get a repeat client be entering Fight or Flight mode and thus acquiring a stress response?

2. If the bodyworker is acquiring a stress response, could they then be sending more blood to their appendages and be preparing to use more muscle effort in their arms and legs (using more appendicular muscles)?

3. If the bodyworker is using more appendicular muscles due to the stress response, can we assume that they will slip into giving a 'hard' massage AND/OR not fully employ proper body mechanics?

KNOWLEDGE OF PROPER BODY MECHANICS

The last piece that affects our body mechanics is the actual knowledge of proper body mechanics being handed down from massage instructor to massage therapy student. There are a lot of instructors who do not know enough about body mechanics and may not be aware of their bodies well enough to instill a proper foundation in their students. Also, some instructors may continue teaching Swedish and Deep Tissue massage in the classic way as it was taught forty or fifty years ago and body mechanics was not greatly emphasized back then. Remember, back then we also had the cultural/societal perception of 'working hard' and putting our 'backs into it'.

Some instructors, not all of course, believe that what they have been taught is gospel and there cannot be another way of doing things. I had to learn that there are a billion variations to the way we work. Not being a large, muscular man I did not have the resources of large amounts of muscle mass to tap into and so I had to find other ways to employ deeper tissue work. It was too much effort for me to muscle it so I had to find other ways to work just as effectively (or more effectively).

The biggest thing that has expanded my knowledge of body mechanics has been working with my students. Being in the lab of the classroom helps me to see how people react to working under the pressure of supervision and expectations. I have tried exercises and experiments that instill the principles of proper body mechanics. It has been through this trial and error that I have found what works and what doesn't work. Teaching this subject in this way has helped me refine my approach to teaching body mechanics not only to beginning students but to advanced bodyworkers.

CONCLUSION

Giving a 'hard' massage and employing improper body mechanics is connected to the Fight or Flight stress response, the way we perceive how society/culture expect us to move, and what our instructors have handed down to us. Working on a client while having the pressure of wanting to do a 'good job' will cause us to 'stress' and use more muscle than necessary and use our bodies in an unsafe manner.

As an educator, I use the term 'muscling it' (as I'm sure other educators do) to describe how some students will employ a lot of muscle action when incorrectly doing 'hard' massage. It's interesting to note that the Fight or Flight response can also be seen as 'muscling it'.

The dark side of this FOF response is that the more a person enters into the Fight or Flight response, the more they are at risk for repetitive strains injuries due to this 'muscling' action. Being injured and not being able to work can lead to its own stressors which essentially create a vicious cycle that ends up looking more like a compounding spiral (see Figure 3).

In my classes, I run a simple exercise. I ask the practicing student to give the receiving student a short massage and I give them a scenario for their day. I tell the practitioner they have just had a fight with their loved one, there's a leak under their kitchen sink, and they just got chewed out by their boss/landlord/friend whoever. The practicing student inadvertently goes into 'hard' massage mode, throwing proper body mechanics out the window while giving their practice massage. The receiving student then gives their feedback. In most cases the feedback centers around the recipient not being able to relax because they felt the practitioner tense up. I then ask the practicing student to take a few full breaths before they work and I attempt to calm them down by offering them a relaxing grounding image (maybe they're on the beach, the warm sun on their face while sipping a relaxing drink with an umbrella in it). Then I tell them to start working on their colleague and they, if they have been previously taught proper body mechanics techniques, will start to employ proper body mechanics. After a few minutes, the receiving student then gives their feedback once more. In this case, very often the recipient states that they felt they could relax more since they felt the practitioner was also more relaxed. Students then switch roles. This exercise is meant to give each student an understanding of the feeling of a 'hard massage' and will keep this as their baseline. They will then use the 'smart massage' model as an option and hopefully it will be the preferred way of working.

Now that we know that this possibility exists, under normal circumstances would we want to massage/work on a client while we are in Fight or Flight mode? Now that we know this stress response affects the way we work, shouldn't we learn how to get ourselves out of Fight or Flight mode and employ proper body mechanics for everyone's sake?

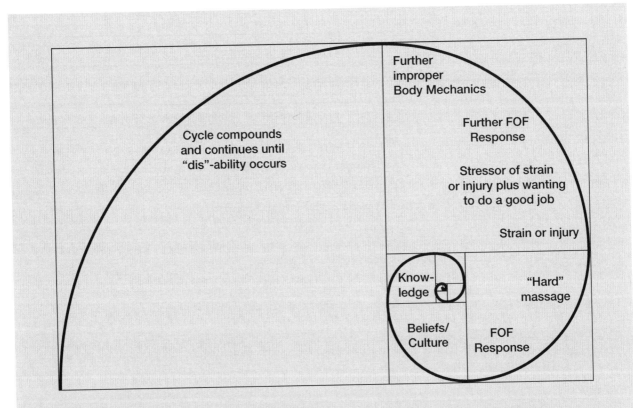

Figure 3. Pictorial representation of the Improper Body Mechanics Theory (with apologies to Fibonacci)

CHAPTER 3:

COUNTERING IMPROPER BODY MECHANICS:

RECOGNITION

I have gone to many spas and done talks to massage therapists there. I have gone to great high-end spas and have met and worked with fantastic bodyworkers. I remember one time at a body mechanics workshop I spoke on everything you have just read. One massage therapist in particular was always shaking her head 'yes'. Whenever I said something she wholeheartedly agreed. When it came time to practice, she went to the table and it was as if she hadn't heard a word I said or was even in the room when I gave my demonstration. I came over and offered a different way of working. She seemed nervous that I singled her out and quickly agreed with me and started to do it the way I showed her. Not a few minutes later I turned to her side of the room and noticed she had gone right back to her old habits.

I wondered what I could do to break this cycle. I went over there and just told her to breathe naturally, to relax her breath, and I offered her a scenario: imagine you are giving a massage on a beach, under a gazebo, this is your last massage of the day and soon you will be having lunch with your friends, sipping on a drink with a paper umbrella in it. She relaxed and started employing better body mechanics.

It was obvious to me that we can counter improper mechanics by not only exploring different ways of working with our bodies but also by exploring the Mastering piece of body mechanics. We must first be aware that improper body mechanics has a root in our FOF response. From that acknowledgement we can overcome improper body mechanics by first addressing our stress response, finding a new way of dealing with our stress, then exploring different techniques that improve our body mechanics. It is this way that we are on our way to making changes permanent and long lasting.

Recognizing Improper Body Mechanics

When I was going through the first piece of my Rolfing® training in Boulder Colorado, I remember doing a practicum and working on some fascia on my classmate's shoulder. He was sitting and I was standing, working over him. I was focused and my intent was very clear. My instructor was coming over in my direction and I was certain she was about to tell me what a great job I was doing but instead she put her hand on my shoulder and I instantly realized that my shoulder was by my ear. I slowly lowered it, embarrassed by my bad body mechanics. I had been a bodyworker for five years at that point and had been teaching for about two years and I had done such a rookie move!

The instructor smiled at me and I sheepishly smiled back. She said, "This is something you're going to be working on for a while."

Sure enough it has been an area (my right shoulder to be specific) where I go to as a check on myself to see if I'm using my body correctly.

I hadn't noticed it at that point. I had always thought my body mechanics were pretty good up to that point and I was disappointed in myself for having done such a beginner's mistake in front of my Rolfing instructor. Looking back, I knew that I was a bit nervous about being in the spotlight (in that particular instance we were working for the sake of being evaluated by the instructors). Being in the spotlight caused me to be nervous and stressed over wanting to impress my instructor, to do a good job in front of them. I allowed this stress response to happen and thus I ended up with a contracted trapezius muscle and raised shoulder, and a possible strain waiting to happen.

I am conveying this story because I want to let you know that bad body mechanics can sometimes be difficult to spot, especially in your own body. Here is a list of things to watch out for in your own body that could be an indicator of improper body mechanics:

1. You're in pain – This could be a possible indicator of improper body mechanics since pain is usually the body's signal that something isn't right. If you are feeling pain only when doing bodywork or if you only get a certain type of pain after doing bodywork, it's time to first get checked out by your physician (in case there might be some RSI symptom or possible nerve injury) and then employ a regimen of bodywork/ grounding/physical therapy that includes an overhaul of your body mechanics.

2. There's constant muscular tension in your body – It's not expected that you will be the perfect Zen master with a fluid like movement of your body but improper body mechanics can start to show itself in the constant contraction of large muscles. For example, do you find yourself with your shoulders up to your ears? Are you grasping muscle tissue? Do you find yourself with your gluteal muscles tightened up all the time? Constant muscular tension is an indicator of a possible FOF stress response.

3. You have an un-human stance – We were meant to move with one foot forward with the whole foot moving along the ground. If you have noticed that your bodywork is having you shuffle around the table like a crab or if you have noticed that you're working with your toes curled up or in, or if you finish your strokes by lifting your foot minus the heel (which stays on the ground) then your body mechanics might need some tweaking. A horse stance is not the universal stance for all massage strokes and should not be deemed as such.

4. You get very tired after a day of work – Yes, we all get tired from doing this type of work. But if you find yourself extra tired after working on one client and you don't feel the slightest bit energized from the great work you and your client did, then it's time to find a possible alternative to working. I gave a body mechanics workshop at a local spa once and one of the bodyworkers contacted me weeks later. She wanted

to tell me that she thought her body mechanics were pretty good to begin with but after taking the workshop, she realized she could change things up. After working for a while with these adjustments, she realized she wasn't as tired as she once was. She had no idea that she didn't have to be as tired as she always was. She accepted a weary body to be the norm from a long day of bodywork (the 'work hard' mentality was dominant with her).

The following is a list of improper body mechanics postures. Perhaps you have done some of these moves yourself. If so, then it's a good thing you've decided to read this book! Please note I don't just show the arms or hands in these moves. Improper body mechanics is neither just hands nor just arms. Improper body mechanics just as proper body mechanics includes the whole body. Improper body mechanics, just as proper body mechanics, is a whole body approach.

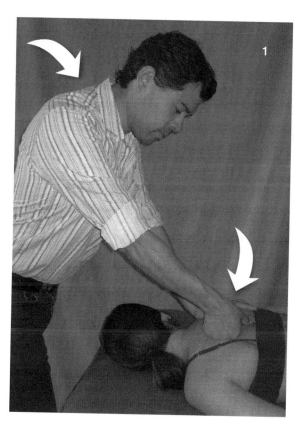 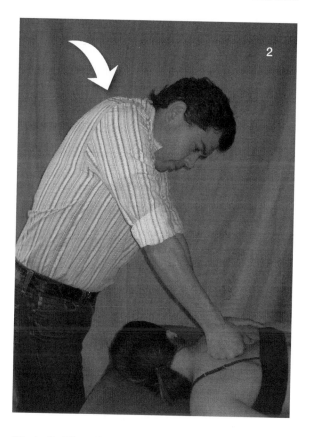

Photo 1: The bent/twisted wrist — This move puts undue strain on the carpal bones and muscles and tendons working to maintain integrity in the wrist. Notice how the right wrist is bent. The energy of the fist is going in a downward direction while the rest of the forearm is putting forth forward energy. Putting your wrist in a manner that is not aligned with the upper bones is equivalent to putting up a column to support a weight and then cutting the column in half and then attempting to brace it with ropes and cables. In the photo my right forearm muscles are working unnecessarily to maintain integrity of the 'column.'

Photo 2: The raised shoulder — Nothing says stress or FOF more than a raised shoulder or shoulders. Here I am depicting a massage therapist with their shoulder up to their ears. This is an over exertion of trapezius muscles, extensors of the forearm and also a contraction of shoulder girdle muscles, low back, and possibly jaw muscles. Eventhough the client might be feeling the sensation of a deep tissue work, the massage therapist is having to work too much to get the desired effect. Eventually the massage therapist will need a massage of their own to work out the tension in their shoulders.

20

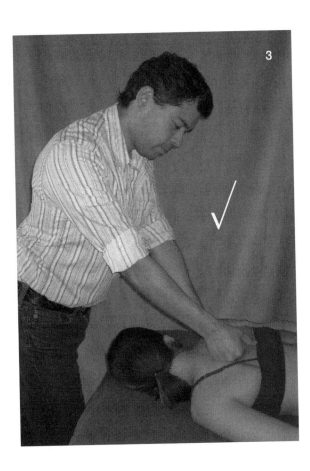

Photo 3: An alternative approach to the above techniques would be to work with lowered shoulders, relaxed upper body, and aligning the joints in the wrist and elbow. Notice there is no unnecessary strain or work. The difference in the forearm muscles between this photo and ones before it is noticeable. The extensors of the forearm are not as engaged as in the previous photos. Less 'muscling!'

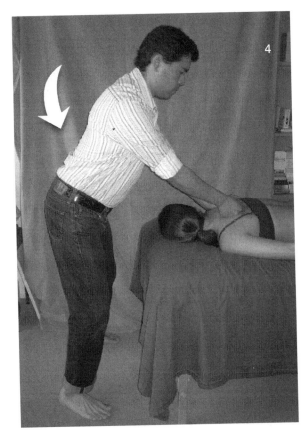

Photo 4: The Horse Stance — Working from a horse stance and attempting to do strokes in a forward and backward manner while in a horse stance is a quick way to put strain on the lower back (see the over lordotic curve occurring in my back). I see a lot of students attempt to perform an effluerage stroke while in horse stance and some tell me they feel they can lean into a client's back that way but how do they pull out of this stroke when they need to? What ends up happening is that the massage therapist would push away from the client and that usually doesn't feel good for the client or, they end up putting one foot in front of another anyway. I sometimes see students practicing this stance and sometimes they modify their body and put one foot in front of the other after being in the horse stance in order to move around. Some practitioners have called that foot in front of the other the Human Stance, I call it the Forward Stance. If we are going to have to put one foot in front of another to move around our client's body, why not stay in that position? My only exception to the forward stance in Swedish massage is when we perform a side to side Petrissage stroke. More on that later.

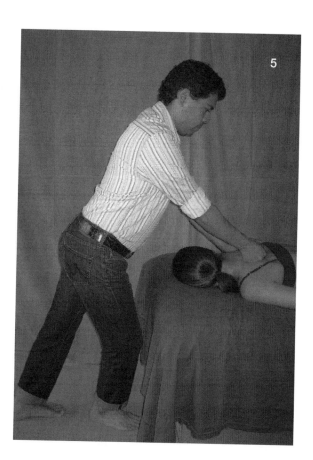

Photo 5: The Off Stance — This stance is when a massage therapist has their feet in a sort of forward stance but the stance is more narrow than the width of their pelvis, creating too narrow a base. It can also happen when one foot is too far away from the other foot as in a lunge. This type of stance does not enable movement and when I see this stance it is indicative of improper body mechanics in the upper body. This stance also indicates that the practitioner may be tapping into a previous resource such as dance or yoga thinking this previous resource will easily transfer into massage. Although dance and yoga are fantastic forms of movement and self-awareness for the body and being, when doing a massage there is now the added component of working with movement and in gravity to facilitate change for the client through manual therapy. For those folks who come with a past movement background I lovingly tell them to prepare to unlearn because their present knowledge may not 100 percent correlate to a Swedish massage or a deep tissue stroke. Notice in the photo that I am almost walking a tightrope and can be easily pushed over.

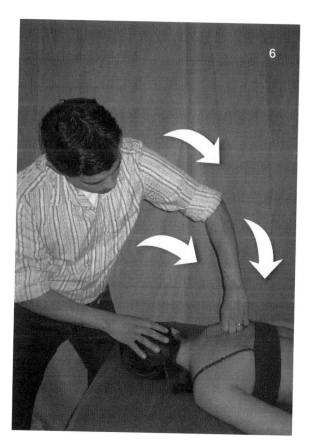

Photo 6: The Wandering Elbow — Whenever I see in an elbow sticking out during a deep tissue stroke I think "strain on the shoulder girdle!" There are a lot of muscles in the shoulder girdle and for a lot of people (especially the muscular ones) it can take a long time before they start to feel the strain of an elbow being out and the whole arm not aligned. When the arm is in this position, there is energy going in many different directions and the muscles, tendons, and ligaments need to work over-time to stabilize the shoulder girdle and create a downward pressure. Note that my humerus is going towards the client's feet while my forearm is going towards the floor. Note also that the hand is starting to get misaligned with the carpal bones.

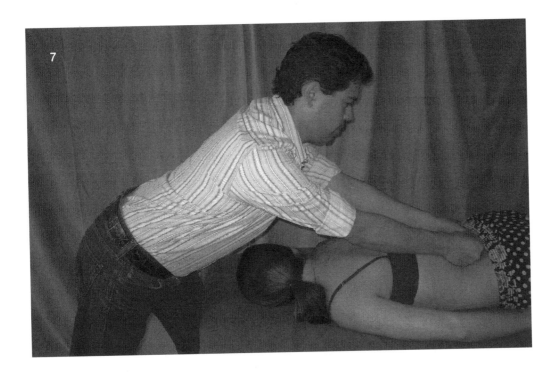

7

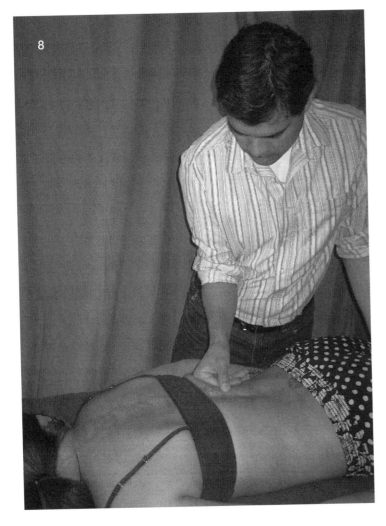

8

Photos 7 & 8: The Proximity Problem — I sometimes see a massage therapist working too close or too far from the body part or client. When the massage therapist works too close, joints need to be bent as a result and strain can occur, throwing proper body mechanics out the window. Usually tendons and ligaments around the bent joint need to take on more strain and usually it ends up being wrist, elbow and/or shoulder. When the massage therapist works too far from the body part I often see them over-reaching and that can lead to possible strain in the back from having to straighten up after the stroke is completed. Since we are all uniquely different with respect to length of arms and size of hands, length of legs, arm reach, etc, the distance benchmark from body part/client to practitioner varies from person-to-person. One technique that works for one person may not work for another person. Notice in the top photo the technique I'm using may actually look very familiar and may look like a technique actually taught by your favorite instructor. The technique, although a good technique to start with gives some students some trouble in the sense that students will try to use it for deeper work and the technique will create undue strain in the body and arm. For this reason, I remind students to use it only for Swedish and to use something else for deeper tissue work.

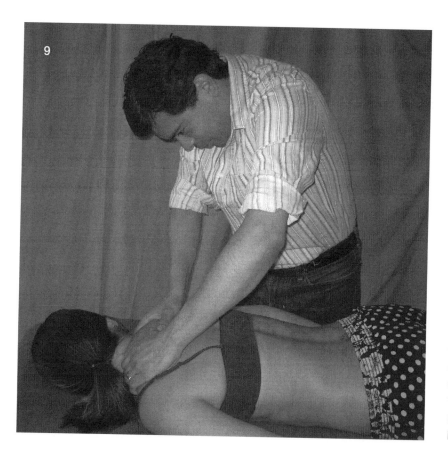

Photo 9: The Hunched Over —
Have you found yourself in this position? Maybe you've wanted to do a great job, impress a client and get that tension out of their shoulders no matter what. And then, ten minutes into it, you find yourself hunched over your client. While you're hunched over you're probably also using primarily your hands and not the whole body. Being hunched over closes out the chest and restricts movement not only within the practitioner but eventually within the client when it comes to having to move the client around (stretches, range of motion movements, etc.). Having a hunched over posture can lead to all sorts of ailments like back strain, hand and wrist strain, and in some cases I have seen massage therapists that hunch over a lot get plantar fasciitis (I have no definite proof there's a connection).

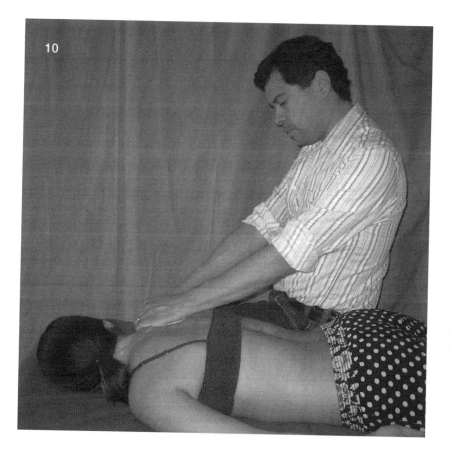

Photo 10: When we examine a hunched over posture, we notice all the anterior flexors (rectus abdominus for example) are in a contracted position, very much like a boxer in a fighting stance. And like a boxer in a fighting stance, a massage therapist being hunched over is also hunched over as a FOF stress response to the stress of wanting to do a good job and impress the client but in effect they massage the person 'strong' or 'hard' and not smart. In the following photo I am offering an alternative to the hunched over position for this particular stroke. Notice I'm leaning back instead of muscling it forward. Leaning back allows me to use my body weight to give a stretch to the trapezius muscles.

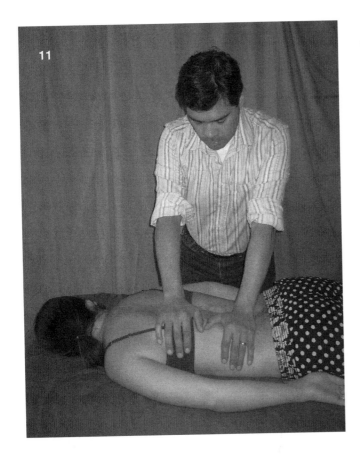

Photos 11, 12, and 13: The "Busy Hands" aka the "Statue" — This happens a lot when I see a massage therapist get caught up in their work, what I will call 'stuck in the lab'. Nothing else seems to move in this massage therapist, they'll stay still as a statue and all I will see moving are their hands. This brings up an analogy told to me long ago. Imagine you have a garden hose in your garden. Let's say you turn on the faucet and see the water coming out of the end of the garden hose. If someone were to ask you, "where is the water originating from?" would you say, "from the end of the garden hose."? No you wouldn't. The water is not originating from the end of the garden hose but from a 'source' (in the case of the water, a reservoir or lake) not possibly seen. The same goes for the 'busy hands' style. The energy/force necessary to create a stroke is not originating from the hands, so why should only the hands move? The hands are actually the same as the end of the garden hose, the end from which the 'water' or energy flows to create the stroke. The spout of the hose, gushing with water is not the source of the water. The source of the water is somewhere else. In this example, we can use it as an analogy for the role of our hands in a massage stroke.

When I see a massage therapist completely stationary, not using their whole body to make a stroke I will say they have 'dropped anchor'. Again, this may have been a way they were taught to massage or maybe an instructor never corrected them but I'm here to say this method of working lays down a foundation for bad habits that might carry on to other parts of their life. If a massage therapist is not used to moving their lower half or their whole body in Swedish, will they be easily convinced to employ their bodies differently in Deep Tissue?

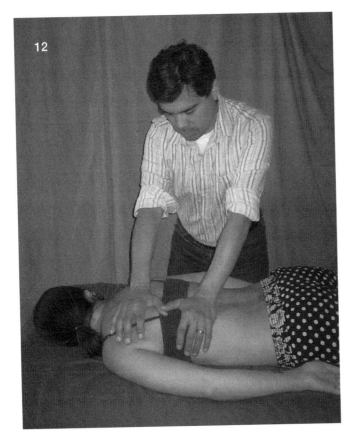

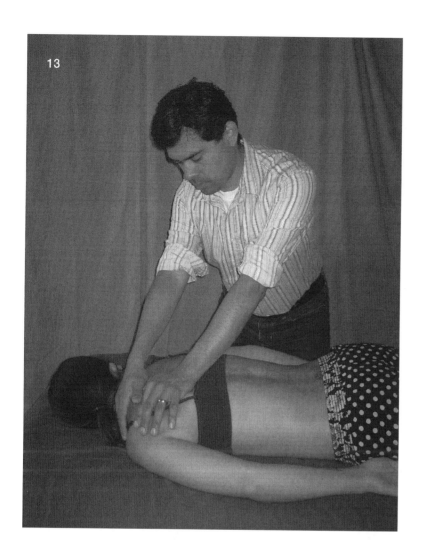

If you've found yourself doing any of the described moves, then it's time to revisit your body mechanics. The first step we will take into employing proper body mechanics is by going into the mind and affecting our stress response. This simple approach has been used by many students with great results. Again, I encourage you to not skip around with this book. Every point brought up here is meant to build on the previous one in order to build a strong foundation in the way you use your body.

CHAPTER 4:

COUNTERING IMPROPER BODY MECHANICS:

GROUNDING PRACTICES

There are various simple, inexpensive and highly effective grounding practices that are useful to reset the nervous system and get the bodyworker out of FOF. These practices positively affect our body mechanics by increasing our level of self awareness, de-stressing us and relieving any muscle strain or tension that may have occurred due to entering FOF and employing improper body mechanics. The following is a brief list of some exercises that I have used and have recommended to my students.

1. Breathwork

Taking some time to breathe fully and intentionally (notice I didn't write 'deeply' as 'fully' I believe is a better adjective to describe the act of filling our lungs with air) goes a long way to calm the nervous system and bring us out of FOF. If you are working at a spa and have back to back to back clients, right before you enter the treatment room, take a couple of full breaths and focus on your self in the present time. If you are seeking more advanced breathwork, one method that

has worked for me is the Yogic breathwork such as Anuloma Viloma, or Alternate Nostril Breathing. I suggest seeking the instruction of a yoga teacher qualified to teach Anuloma Viloma. Alternatively, a simple breathing exercise such as the following can also help:

Close your eyes and be either lying down or sitting and rest your hands at your sides or rest them right above your navel and sternum. Start by focusing on how you are currently breathing. Notice where your breath is going to. Are you breathing more into your belly or into your chest? Did you find that you may have actually been holding your breath? If you find yourself breathing into one area more than another (belly or chest), whichever one you are currently breathing into, imagine yourself breathing into both the belly and chest. Do not increase your rate of breath to the point of hyper ventilation. This may be different than other breathing techniques you may have practiced, and is called Full Body Breathing or what some people call

Baby Breathing (look at babies when they breathe, it seems their whole body is taking in the breath). Breathing and being mindful of the whole system has the added benefit of quickly relaxing me and 'resetting' my nervous system (If I happen to find myself in FOF). Do this a couple of times before a session and make a mental note as to whether it helped you or not. This technique can be expanded upon and you can imagine breathing into any other body part in addition to the belly or chest.

b. Another method of breathwork is to breathe and count as your exhale. Before a session and before entering the treatment room, breathe fully into your belly. Take a brief pause between inhale and exhale. As you breathe out, slowly and quietly count to one. As you continue this process, count "two" with the next exhale, and so on. You will notice that you will be breathing slower, you'll be more relaxed, and your muscular tension will have diminished. If you find yourself stressed about something (again, the perpetual desire to do a good job) make a note as to whether that stress went away with this technique.

2. Meditation Practice

Having a meditation practice helps tremendously to ground and center the bodyworker and improve body mechanics. How so? Meditating allows you to better deal with the everyday stresses that occur in life. Being able to do so allows you to respond to them without a FOF stress response. This in turn prevents the FOF stress response from happening in the first place and from affecting muscle contraction, or 'muscling' it. Thus, overall body mechanics are not adversely affected during a bodywork session. In the beginning of my practice the bodywork seemed to be the actual meditation for me (in addition to being the work I got paid to do). I was able to work with clients and focus on the work, not focus with intensity but focus and be present with what I was doing at that particular point in time. If my mind wandered I allowed it to wander, was conscious of the wandering but then I brought it back to the present moment into the work that I was doing. Maybe because the work was so new to me and I did not have the experience of having to be present all the time (think about it, when you weren't doing bodywork and had another job, how present were you throughout the day, how often did you actually seek distraction in order not to be present?) that bodywork was a meditative practice for me.

Now with a practice that is full and other projects taking up more of my time I feel that in addition to the bodywork itself, there are other practices that can and need to be done to achieve grounding. Simple things such as walking and breathing or being aware of your breath as you're walking or alternating your breath to match certain steps are different ways of mastering the mind and are meditative practices. Personally, mediation takes on many variations. I can spend long quiet minutes while having a cup of tea and cake while savoring the flavors and to me that is a meditation. Beethoven was famous for taking long walks in nature and making notes in a notebook during these walks. If you want to follow a specific structured meditative practice there are many methods available. Transcendental Meditation, Zen Meditation, or to follow what Swami Vishnu Devananda calls the 12 principles are all ways of meditation. Below is a simple and effective meditation that I follow:

a. **Self Awareness Meditation** – This is another meditation method that helps to tap into the awareness of your body while also releasing body tension: Start by noticing your own breath. Notice where it goes in your body (belly or chest). After a few breaths, start to bring awareness to your feet. Start bringing awareness to the soles of your feet and notice without attempting to change anything if there's any tension there. Imagine your breath going down into your feet with every inhale. As you continue this process, notice if the tension in that area dissipates. From your feet you can slowly move your attention/intention further up your body to your knees, thighs, pelvis, torso, arms, shoulders, neck, face and head. Essentially this method can be used to bring attention, breath, intention, and tension relief to any area of the body. In my practice, I also tend to meditate when I'm in a particular stretch or stretched position. I am focused on being aware of a particular body part and what it's doing/how it's positioned. It is important that as you are focused on a particular area and you might be experiencing tension there not to focus on that area with any goal, expectation or judgment.

3. Preparation/Reset Ritual Before And After a Session

Professional athletes have a ritual or protocol that they practice before and after a game. Some type of visualization exercise, tapping of the feet, shaking off of the legs; something that helps to focus and mentally prepare for the event that will unfold before them. We as bodyworkers also use our bodies as athletes do; so should we not also mentally prepare for our work? Before a session, I will wash my hands and do a light warm up exercise or envisioning exercise. After the session I do a light stretch and wash my hands to keep my self grounded and focused on the rest of my day. I open the windows and prepare the

room for the next client. I suggest if you don't have a preparation ritual to adopt something to help you re-focus and ground yourself. This will go a long way to put you in the present and give you an awareness of where you are in your body and thus where you want to be with your body mechanics. These movements are seen as physical warm-up exercises but they can also be seen as a way of dealing with a stress response in the same way athletes could be dealing with the pressure of performance.

4. Shaking It Off

As many of you know that have lived with pets, they are a special gift and enrich our lives immensely. My wife and I were lucky to have had eleven years with a special little being named Maggie. Maggie was a wee puppy when we met her at the pound. A little ball of fur, she was trembling in the corner of the kennel as all the other dogs were jumping around for our attention. Needless to say, we chose her (or she chose us, however you want to see it). Having a little kennel trauma, she grew up not exactly getting along with other dogs but easily charmed any human she encountered. On walks she would sometimes growl or bark at other dogs. After her 'arguments' she would trot off and shake herself vigorously. At first I thought it was funny but I soon realized she was actually shaking off the experience! After speaking with a trainer, I was told Maggie entered FOF mode and in order to 'reset' her nervous system and not stay in FOF mode she literally shook it off. I haven't accumulated data on whether or not humans do this similar action to reset their nervous system but something I find interesting is that boxers right before a fight will jump up and down and shake their arms and head. Is this part of their warm up or meant for something else? Could it be meant to shake off the pre fight jitters? I have tried it myself after a full day or in between sessions and it's helped! If at the very least shaking it off helps to distract oneself from the tension or stress at hand, I would suggest trying it in private and seeing if it helps you.

Check Your Body Mechanics, Folks

Grounding practices helps body mechanics in that it resets the nervous system, grounds the individual and sets a firm foundation where a grounded individual can begin to question the cultural perceptions of 'working hard' and begin the unlearning of having to 'muscle' it. From there, the individual can be exposed to a different option of working, one where movement and gravity help the practitioner create the strokes rather than sheer muscle. If you have tried the meditation and grounding techniques and still find yourself feeling strain or feeling like there is possibly an easier way to work then you might be in need of revising the way you work, your actual body mechanics.

At this point I have been teaching beginning Swedish massage for about five years. Once, during a class I was looking around and noticed a raised shoulder over here, muscling techniques over there, and an un-human stance further down the room. Instead of going to each student individually I tried something different. I made an announcement during the class: "Please check your body mechanics folks."

Easily, the raised shoulder came down, someone else put themselves in a forward stance and another student stopped muscling through their techniques. The students already knew what the proper body mechanic techniques were but they just needed to be gently reminded. From there I started using a very simple exercise: I would tell my students to briefly imagine as if they were looking at themselves work for a moment and see themselves from five feet away. As they see themselves work, I ask them to examine their body mechanics. In doing so, they would correct themselves or make any adjustments. It was the equivalent of an out of body experience method of correcting body mechanics! If this technique is too abstract for some students, I would walk around the room with a large full-length mirror and have them look at themselves in the mirror. They have already been taught proper body mechanics and now they can see themselves do it. This helps them check to see if they were employing the techniques that they were taught.

This exercise helps bodyworkers see the bigger picture (figuratively and literally in the mirror!) and helps them not only to be more aware of their bodies but also find out there's another way, a more effective way of using their bodies. Before you can check your body mechanics during an out of body experience, it's imperative to instill proper awareness exercises and then proper body mechanics techniques.

Mastering Body Mechanics

Chapter 5:

The Beginnings of Proper Body Mechanics:

Awareness Exercises

Before I cover the principles of body mechanics I first take my students through some awareness exercises. These awareness exercises help to physically familiarize the student with the principles that lead to proper body mechanics. I believe the principles for proper body mechanics differ between Swedish and Deep Tissue massage modalities, and I believe they differ enough to be addressed separately so I teach slightly different awareness exercises for each.

Awareness Exercises for Swedish and Western Massage Therapy

In teaching a Swedish or Western Massage therapy class, a proper foundation of body mechanics should be first priority. Before we go into the stances and the proceeding movements and strokes, we need to understand that Swedish is meant as a relaxing and therapeutic modality. It is not meant to be a deep tissue modality and because of this the body mechanics for Swedish are particular and unique from other modalities (Shiatsu, Sports Massage, etc.). It is not meant to work on deeper layers of muscle

tissue in the way that Deep Tissue does so the body mechanics will be different.

The Main Principle of Swedish Body Mechanics

To start off, we address the main principle behind body mechanics for Swedish massage therapy: Movement. In order to have proper body mechanics for this modality, we need to move effectively, efficiently and safely around the client and/or table and have the means to do so. Following and understanding this thinking will help the practitioner avoid injury and give a massage that is enjoyable and therapeutic. In order to move properly and to efficiently deliver the stroke, we start with the proper way to stand, our stance.

The Stance - When we develop as babies, it is common knowledge that most of us first learn to sit, crawl, stand, and then walk. Placing our legs and feet under our bodies gives us stability and help us for the next step, literally and figuratively. In its very basic form (I am completely oversimplifying it and I'm sure someone who studies Kinesiology would have a lot more to say about this subject than I do) when we learn to walk, we begin by placing one foot in front of another. We learn that not putting our foot forward (as we are intentionally placing ourselves in an unbalanced position in the forward direction) will bring us into off balance in a way that would make us fall flat on our face.

Since we naturally avoid that, we instinctively then keep putting one foot in front of the other.

Walking forward then is a form of controlled forward 'off-balance' or a controlled example of the creation of kinetic energy in the forward direction. So, now we know walking forward produces forward energy. Staying still with both feet planted under your body does not have the benefit of creating this type of energy.

Let's keep that in mind as we proceed with the following exercise that I have my students do in class.

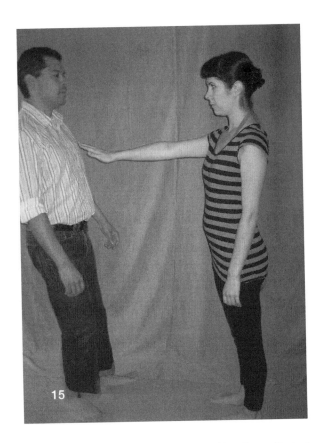

Photo 14: Have two students stand in front of each other. Each will be standing with both feet in a normal standing posture. Their feet should not be wider than their hips. This could be called the Horse Stance and is meant to be a firm, stable stance in many martial arts. The problem with this stance is that it doesn't completely adhere by the principle of body mechanics for Swedish massage which is 'movement'. I say doesn't completely because it can be used to some extent as will be shown later.

Photo 15: One student (student A) will gently but sufficiently push the other student (student B) on the sternum in order to bring them off balance (falling backward). The student doing the pushing will realize that it doesn't take much of a push in order to bring the other student off balance. This is because with both feet firmly planted underneath your body you are off balance in the forward and backward direction (along the sagittal plane). Even if a student resists the gentle push (as I've seen some do in class) I remind them they are still off balance in this position as I gently give them a push from their T1-T2 area towards me and they move off balance in the forward direction.

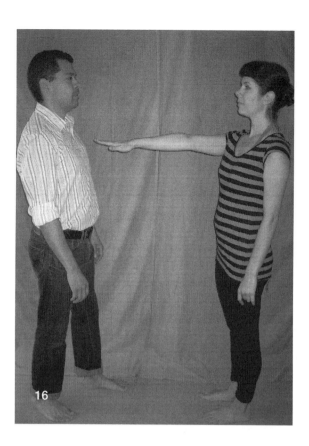

Photo 16: Student B will then avoid falling by placing one foot backward. They have now been forced to go into the Forward Stance from the Horse Stance. This is a clear indicator that what we will call the Horse Stance is an off balance stance when confronted with a forward oncoming kinetic energy. It is also an indicator that the Horse Stance may not be the proper stance when creating a forward kinetic energy (as in moving forward and backward of your own accord).

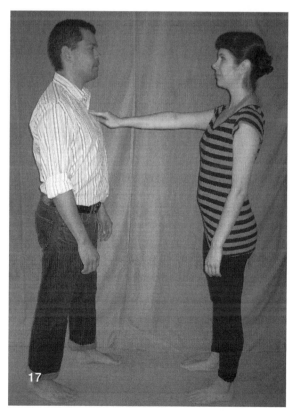

Photo 17: Now repeat the exercise as before but this time have Student B keep one foot forward at a comfortable distance (the feet should still be hip width apart). Again, have student A use the same amount of previous pressure and push Student B in the same location (sternum) and pushing in the same direction. The result is that Student B will not be off balance and almost fall backward. Instead, Student B will be stable. The conclusion? A forward foot posture (the Forward Stance) is more stable than a Horse Stance when we are experimenting with kinetic energy in the sagittal plane.

The Stance – Forward Energy

Now, before we create a stroke on a client, whether it be an effleurage or cross fiber stroke or friction stroke, we need to understand that the hands or forearm are the end point where we visibly see the stroke materialize but it is not the location where the stroke originates. Imagine the garden hose image previously mentioned in Part I. As I mentioned before, the hands are the end product, or the end of the garden hose, not the source of the massage stroke. The source of the stroke in this case is the rest of the body, or as some would think, the feet and lower body. I tend to think that the source of the stroke can be seen as beyond the body itself and can originate in the mind and physically manifest in the whole body and eventually be seen/felt in the hands, soft fist, or elbow, etc.

For this reason, the hands are not the source so they are not meant to grasp, grab, or over exert muscle to create a stroke. Again, the force of the stroke and the energy behind the massage stroke comes from our stance and our use of movement and energy. We find this out by a step by step process, beginning with playing with energy in the Forward Stance.

Moving Forward from the Forward Stance

Now that we know that standing with one foot forward gives you a more balanced stance in the forward direction, let's play with this new way of working. The following photos show stills of movement in the Forward Stance but as I've mentioned before, they do not show the sense of movement.

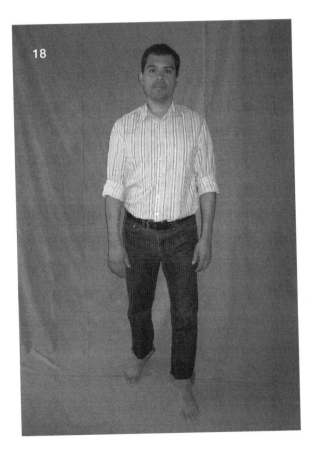

Photo 18: With one foot forward, shift your weight to your front foot and then to your back foot. Imagine you are kelp in the ocean, moving forward and backward with the steady rhythmic movement of the ocean. You will feel the kinetic energy from the shifting of your weight as you sway to and fro. Try this for a minute and sit with the feeling of having your mass moving forward and backward. This is where the energy that travels up to your arms and 'out' your hands comes from.

Photos 19, 20, 21, 22 (next page): This kinetic energy is the energy that is expressed as an effleurage or cross fiber stroke through the hands. In Photo 19 I am in a Forward Stance. In Photo 20, I lean back, putting more weight on my back foot. In Photo 21 I am creating kinetic energy by leaning forward. I then return to the normal stance in Photo 22. Now, in this sequence my arms are up and I am mimicking an effleurage stroke. As I move my weight back and forth I can feel the energy from the movement translate into the effleurage. I would not be able to do this as effectively if I was in the Horse Stance. In fact, attempting to create forward kinetic energy in the horse would cause me to get off balance and I would have to put one foot forward in order to prevent from falling on my face!

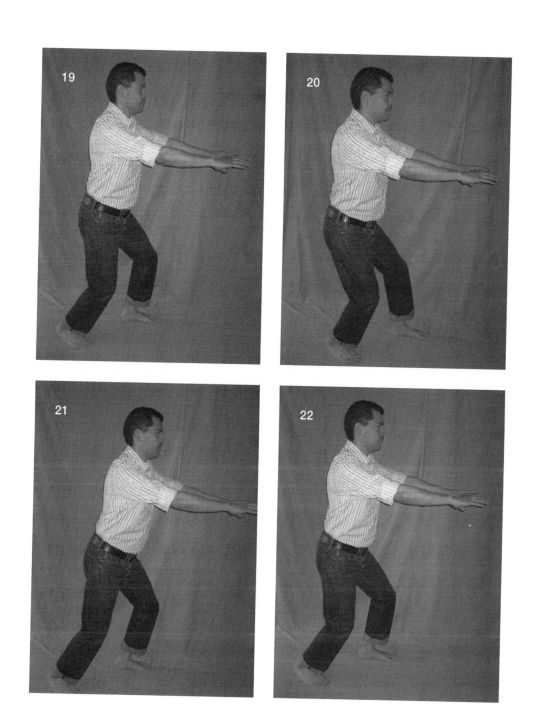

Notice how easy it is to perform this stroke and how you don't have to effort as much. If you weren't moving like this before you might be thinking, "moving this way makes my work so much easier!"

And there's a key thought, we get so used to having to 'work hard' that we sometimes don't realize there's an easier, more effective way of working.

This is the proper use of body mechanics for the effleurage, moving with ease and not with unnecessary exertion. A well known Brazilian Jiu-Jitsu competitor Marcelo Garcia once said (I'm paraphrasing here), "Jiu-Jitsu is not about what is difficult, it's about what is simple". The same can be said for performing a Swedish massage.

Moving Side to Side
in Swedish Massage Therapy

Standing with one foot forward works when we are directing our energy forward but what about when the body's kinetic energy needs to move side to side as in a Swedish Petrissage stroke? In this case the horse stance or having your feet planted under your self is a more effective stance to produce this type of stroke.

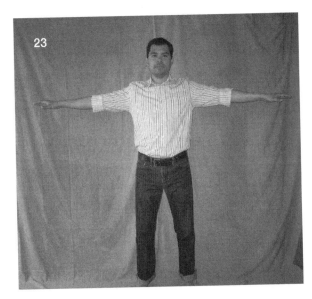

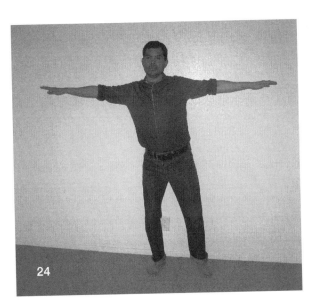

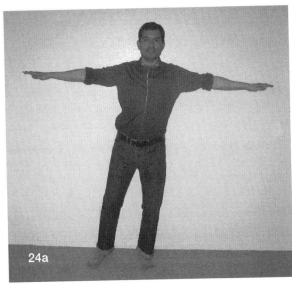

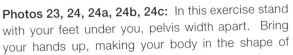

Photos 23, 24, 24a, 24b, 24c: In this exercise stand with your feet under you, pelvis width apart. Bring your hands up, making your body in the shape of a "T". In this stance, shift your weight from your right foot to the left foot. As you're moving your body weight side to side notice how it feels to move it side to side. If done correctly, you will end up bending your knees to take on the weight of your body as in Photos 24 and 24a. That force you feel is what creates the petrissage stroke as you shift your weight from one side to another. Your hands will eventually follow and translate that force to create the stroke on your client. Notice in photos 24b and 24c I'm moving

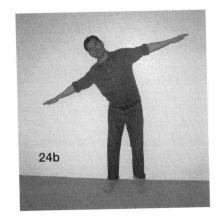

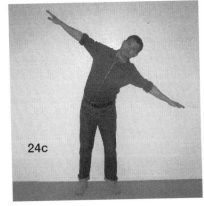

my body incorrectly. This stroke is not created by me bending my upper body from side to side. This creates strain in the low back and actually shuts off the lower half of the body to movement. Doing this sets up a bad habit for future movements and doesn't coincide with our previous premise of Swedish massage strokes being created by the whole body.

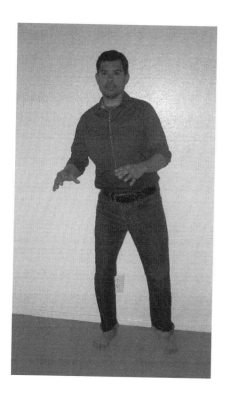 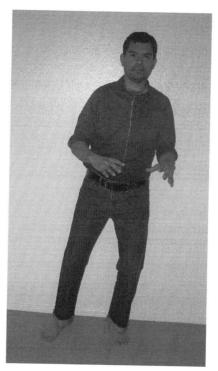

Photos 25, 25a: In these photos you can see how the exercise can transform into a petrissage stroke. My body weight is shifting side to side and now my hands are in the form of a petrissage stroke. Notice again how the stroke is created by movement, a principle of Swedish massage body mechanics. The petrissage stroke is not created by just my hands or just by my upper body but by my whole body. If you find yourself not using your whole body to create this stroke, you could be employing improper body mechanics. Do a check-in with your body to see if you can discover why you're not using your whole body. Does something hurt when you attempt to move?

The previous photos represent just two of the five basic strokes in Swedish. The other three classically are: Tapoutment, Cross Fiber, and Vibration. Other strokes may be taught under the Swedish Massage umbrella. Although I have not shown photos for the other strokes, the movements for them are either the same or slight derivatives of the forward energy or the side by side movement exercises.

Sometimes telling a massage therapy student that movement is the main principle in this modality is not enough information for them. I have been taught and have seen some fantastic instructors use a list of techniques that help massage students remember the main principle. Some of the techniques I have seen are:

1. Keep your chest out

2. Don't drop your head

3. Keep your pelvis aligned in the direction that you're moving

4. Stay behind your tool (in this case, the hand(s) that are doing the stroke)

5. Keep your wrists at a comfortable 45 degree angle

Notice this short list of techniques all support the main principle I have previously described: *we need to move effectively, efficiently and safely around the client or table and have the means to do so.*

We cannot move properly or safely if we have our head dropped or if our chest is sunken in (as seen when we have not straightened our backs). All great techniques for Swedish massage currently being used have one thing in common: They are all encouraging the student to move sufficiently, efficiently, and safely.

Table Height

No good book on body mechanics would be complete without addressing table height. Table height is not an evolution where one day you find the ultimate table height. Table height is a process. It will move up and down throughout your career. In the beginning when I went through school I was given a rough basic guide on determining table height. This is the old stand by: drag your knuckles along the table and if your knuckles barely scrape the table, you have a proper table height. I have debated whether I should even discuss this method as I don't like it and I don't teach it at all. This method will only serve the student for a brief period of time (maybe for as long as the first class). Instead, what I recommend is getting a person on the table and checking for the appropriate angle of your wrists. As I've stated before, make sure the wrists are comfortable at a 45 degree angle. This guide is great for Swedish work. When we get to deep tissue, table height takes on a different dimension. Also keep in mind that putting someone on the table will give you a rough estimate as no two people are alike in size. Some clients may be thicker/bigger than others.

What if you're working at a spa and your client has already gotten on the table and you don't have away to adjust? As I have found in my practice, I can sometimes negate bad table height by getting on the table either in sitting or standing. I've worked in the spa world for a long time and know to check in with the client before sitting or getting on the table. If you have an electric or hydraulic table, even better! As a Rolfer, I will often work with my client while I am sitting or standing on the table. I use the table as a tool and an aide. As a teacher once told me, "the table is your friend". If we understand that we can use the table as a helper, we can see it as a way of doing better work rather than an obstacle that needs to be dealt with. In the proceeding photos I will point out what I am doing as far as specific work but I will also point out when I am using the table to make the work easier for me, while still being effective.

CHAPTER 6:

BODY MECHANICS FOR SWEDISH & WESTERN MASSAGE THERAPY

The following group of photos is a collection of Swedish massage strokes taken and done on different parts of the body to illustrate the proper use of body mechanics. The strokes are laid out in the form of how they may look on different body parts. The most ideal way to learn proper body mechanics is in live action, to be able to see the movements, but my hope is that in looking at these photos and reading the descriptions you can capture the essence of proper body mechanics. Again, my suggestion is to use this book in workshop form with two other people. Have one person attempt the stroke while another colleague explains what is going on in the photo by reading the description of the photo and the third colleague is the recipient. Keep in mind the purpose of the photo is not to completely dictate how your body should be. Your body will be different than mine and attempting to totally mirror me will discount the beautiful way your body is able to move and adapt. Instead, see the photos as a guideline and an illustration of the application of the principles previously described. If used that way and if the description is read and understood in the same way, then maximum benefit and the true message behind the book will be obtained.

What does it feel like to employ proper body mechanics?

Sometimes it's necessary to understand that proper body mechanics will actually feel different than anything else. Here's a brief list of what I have heard students say after they realize a more efficient way of working:

1. This is so much easier

2. I don't feel like I have to work as 'hard'

3. I'm not as tired after the end of my day

4. I don't feel my (fill in your favorite strained body part here) is as strained as before

40

Photo 26: This is the initial effleurage stroke. This initial stroke is meant to introduce yourself to the client and to apply oil/lotion and finally to assess and discern any areas of tightness. It starts at the top of the client's shoulders. Some things to note:

1. My back is pretty straight

2. I am in the Forward Stance

3. My shoulders are relaxed and low

4. My wrists are not compressed or strained

Photo 27: Keeping the back straight (but still keeping my lumbar curve), the movement starts as I begin to lean forward. As I am leaning forward, my back is not bent inward and my legs are taking on any additional stress. This allows me to move easier, my head is up and my feet are relaxed, no toe curling or balancing on a heel, just a relaxed leaning.

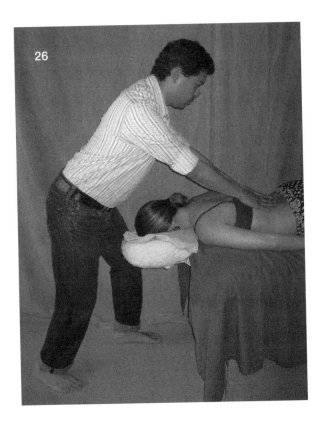

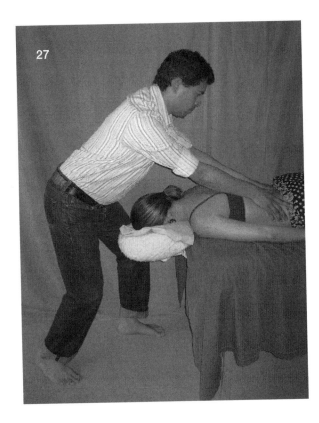

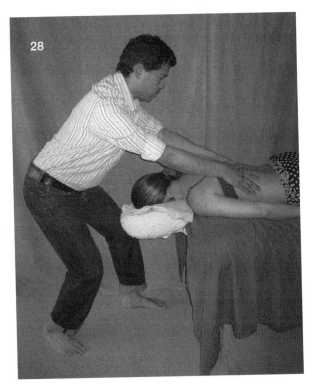

Photo 28: If the client's torso is particularly long (or at least longer than yours), move off to the side to avoid improper body mechanics. Another way to avoid straining the back or lifting from the back is to drop your pelvis to bring the pelvis more underneath your own head and in effect bring the hands back to the upper part of the client's back.

1. Back is still straight versus in a "C" curve

2. Shoulders are still relaxed

In this photo the client is feeling the stroke come from my whole body as opposed to just the hands

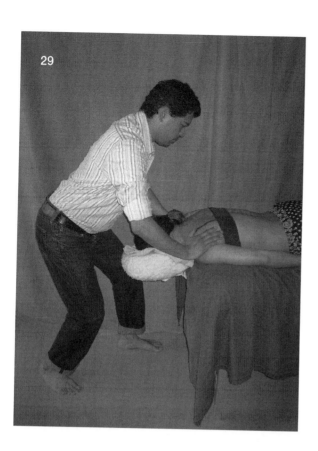

Photo 29: As I'm getting ready to finish off the stroke, I am now moving forward and including the shoulders. Although my wrists may look compressed, there is no pressure on them as this stroke is meant to be a light stroke. I am moving forward and it's easy for me since I'm in the Forward Stance. The elbows are out but it's only because my arms are moving and the arms are moving as a result of my lower body moving. The stroke becomes a whole body stroke.

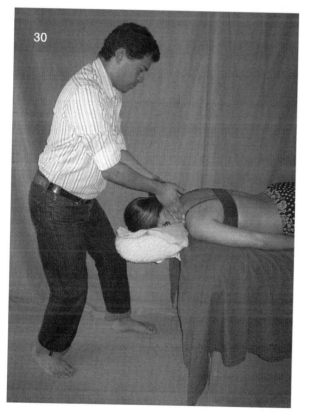

Photo 30: Finishing the initial effleurage with a slow stroke on the neck. I am standing up and moving from my legs. My back is still straight and I move to the client's neck by moving my legs, not from lifting my shoulders.

42

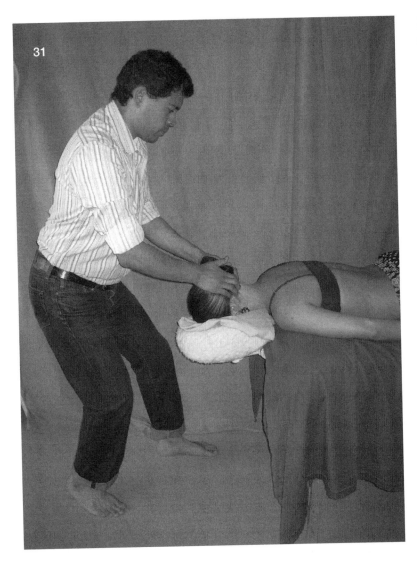

Photo 31: The stroke ends at the client's occiput. Still in the forward stance, I move back and put more weight on my back leg. My feet are still positioned firmly on the floor, my heel is not my only point of contact nor are my toes off the ground. My head is not dropped and I have not sunken in my chest.

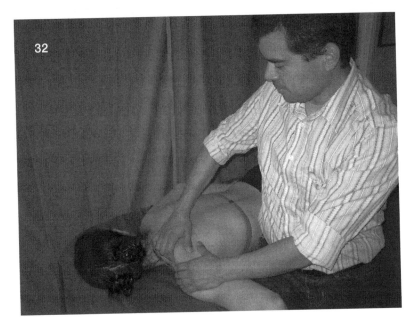

Photo 32: In this petrissage, I am sitting on the table and am massaging the client's upper trapezius. The movement of side to side is still there even though I am sitting. In this case, my upper body is moving toward the client's right then towards the left, still maintaining the image of moving like kelp in the ocean.

1. My head is up

2. I'm not hunched over the client

3. I'm using the table by sitting on it (as the saying goes, "The table is my friend!")

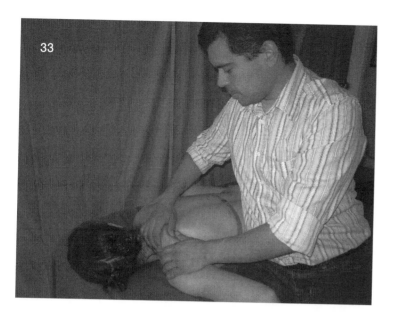

Photo 33: In the following photo I am moving in the other direction to complete the petrissage. Although it may look like the stroke is primarily coming from the thumbs, it's actually the whole body that is creating the stroke. If I was only using thumbs, I can assure you my posture would eventually resemble more of a C curve and my head would drop.

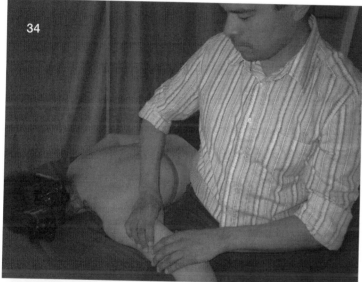

Photos 34 and 35: The same petrissage can be used in this position to work on the triceps. In this case I place the client's arm over my leg making it easier to massage the triceps. The following two photos show the movement back and forth of my body as I create the stroke. Not seen in the photo is my left leg which is out to the side in such a way as to give me stability and support while I am still moving in an easy rhythm, again, my whole body is involved in the stroke. Notice my shoulders are relaxed and even though elbows are out, there is no stress on them since there is no downward pressure, only side to side movement in this stroke.

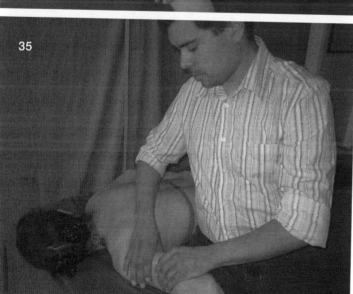

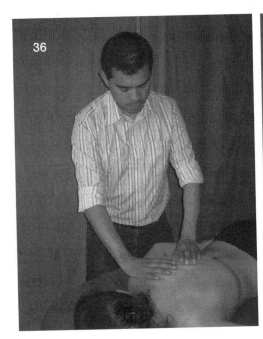
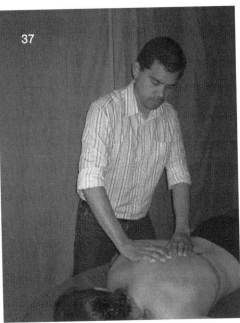

Photos 36 and 37: In this set of photos, I am performing a petrissage on the side of the ribs. I am petrissaging from the same side of the ribs I am on. I am doing this petrissage from a standing position so I will be using the same body mechanics as displayed in the Horse Stance. My knees are bending as I move side to side and I am not 'muscling' it in my hands, my hands are following the side to side movement of my whole body.

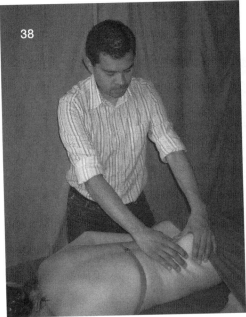
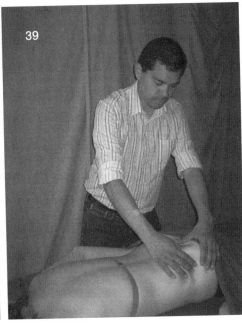

Photos 38 and 39: Here I am displaying a petrissage on the gluteal muscles. In order to do this stroke across the table, the table height and the client's proportions need to be such that I am not leaning forward. An electric table in this instance would help you adjust the height quickly. Notice my knees are bent and I am focused on not straining my back. Also, my arms are out and shoulders relaxed, they are not scrunched up. Finally, my pelvis is parallel to the side of the table and not pitched forward (in anterior tilt). For this and all strokes, the stroke is coming from me moving my whole body. If any strain is felt in the low back, then don't pursue this stroke. Move to the other side of the table and petrissage from there.

Photos 40 and 41: In a cross fiber stroke on the back, I am in a Forward Stance and my whole body moves along a vertical axis that is parallel to my spinal column. When thinking about where the energy is coming from that creates this stroke, it's important to think that it could be coming from a whole body-mind dynamic. Meaning, the mind is aware of making the stroke from a whole body perspective (simply, I'm imagining rotating along a vertical axis) and the body will follow suit by

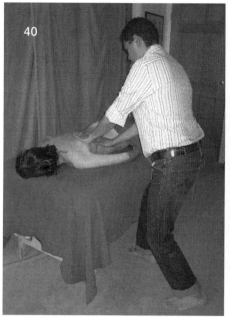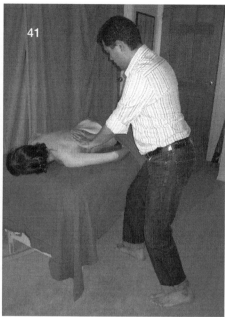

shifting weight, rotating hips and moving arms and hands anterior and posterior to create a cross fiber action! Notice I am in forward stance and not in a Horse stance. Also notice my chest is open and my head is not dropped. The stroke is not coming from arms or shoulders as they are the ending point for the stroke and I am not over extending my arms or hands (if I did, I wouldn't be able to move as efficiently or as safely as possible).

Photos 42 and 43: A tapoutement can be performed easily in the forward stance. Although it could also be performed in a horse stance, I choose the forward stance because if I were to move around the table (which I will most likely do during a massage) I will need to put one foot forward anyway. Notice my legs are bent and I'm bouncing up and down with my soft fists to create percussion on the client's back. My back is straight, my transverse abdominus muscles are engaged and the movement is coming from my whole body

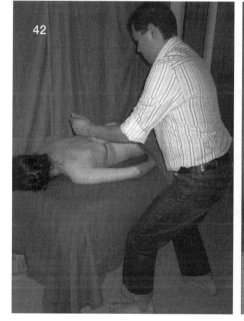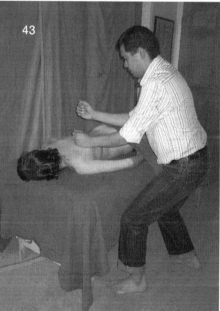

moving up and down rather than my back bending forward. Finally, my feet are flat on the ground, no curled toes or heel or toes off the ground.

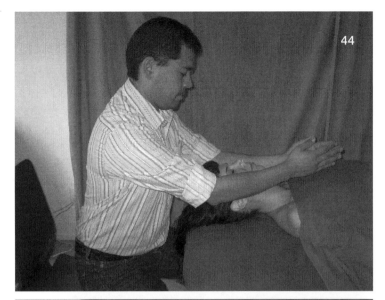

Photos 44 and 45: During a full effleurage on the face, I lean back to allow the whole forearm to effleurage the face. The table height is such that my arms can relax on the table without me having to bend forward. The distance between me and the table is a comfortable one, I am not bending over the client's face or right up close to her head. I am rocking forward and backward on my ischial tuberosities. I imagine my tuberosities are like feet on the floor except they are on the chair. This allows me to keep the rhythm of movement even though I'm sitting. Leaning back allows me to effleurage the client's face without having to raise my shoulders. In this sitting position, I still have one foot forward.

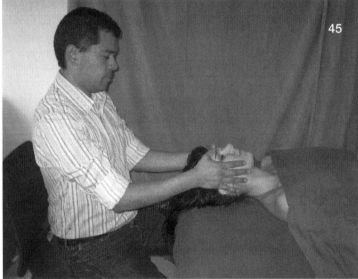

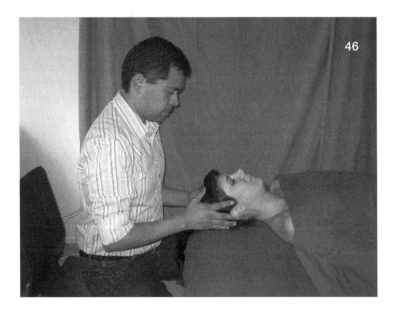

Photo 46: Starting with the top of the head I am using my thumbs to press along the client's head while employing my upper body weight. I make sure I am moving with my whole body forward and backward. Instead of using muscle, the act of me leaning forward is creating the compression. When I teach this technique I usually like to tell my students to pretend they are kelp in the ocean and mimic that slow rhythmic movement of the kelp. This takes strain away from the thumbs and hands. Notice my fingers are relaxed and not stiff and even though I'm sitting, I still have one foot/leg forward as if in Forward Stance.

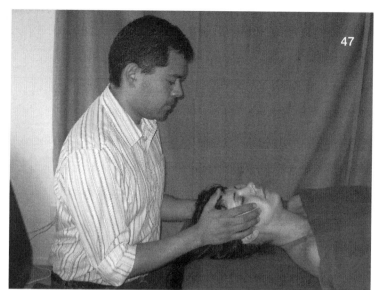

Photos 47 and 48: Using my whole body, I am doing circles on the masseter area. My fingers are moving in a circular fashion and my whole upper body is moving forward and backward, creating the stroke in the same fashion as before. I'm not slumped in my chair and I keep the image in my mind of moving like kelp. The same movement can be done on the sub-occipital muscles. Instead of having to grab or squeeze the head, I am instead using movement and kinetic energy to create the circular movement on the occiput.

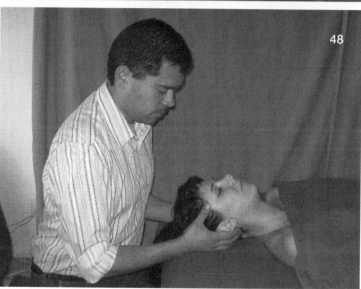

48

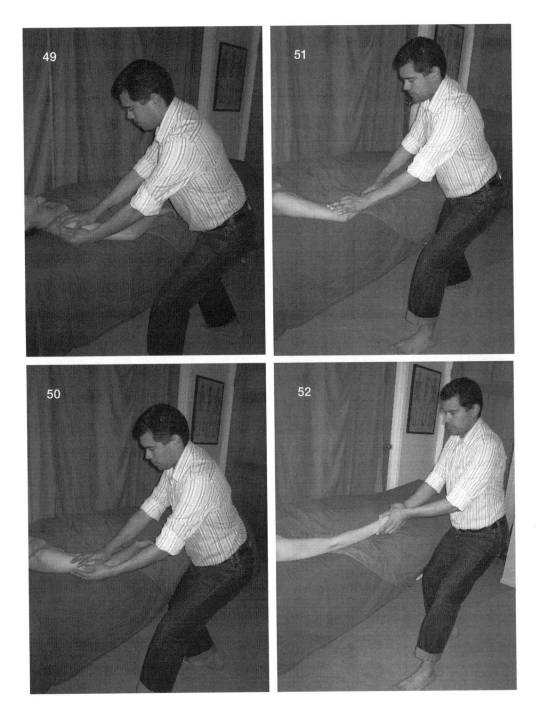

Photos 49, 50, 51, and 52: In this version of an effleurage on the arm, I start by moving backwards, from the shoulder and ending with the hand. I start in the Forward Stance and although you might notice in this photo that this stance is a bit narrow I am relying on the table for some stability. The table is still my friend! Initially, I start with more weight on my forward foot but eventually place more weight on my back foot as my body, arms, and hands move back, creating the stroke that goes down the arm. As I get to the elbow, I take half a step back and repeat the process with the forearm. If necessary, I take another micro step back to finish off with the hands. Notice my back is straight in the whole movement. My hands are relaxed and there is no 'muscling' in them.

In the last photo, I am working the hands exclusively. Working on the hands I will tend to move back and forth, using the forward stance to produce a gentle tug on the metacarpals and phalanges. This slow rhythmic movement has the pleasant side effect of gently pulling on their arm and also stretching the upper trapezius. Note my shoulders are not up by my ears and my elbows are in, creating a straight line in my arms.

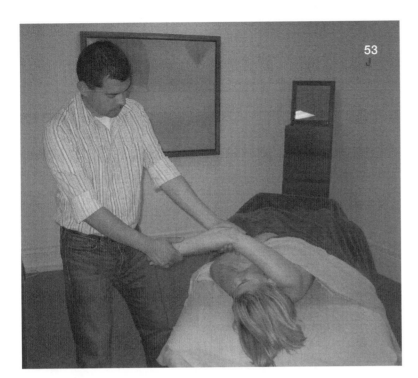

Photo 53: Although not a Swedish massage stroke, this stretch illustrates how to properly employ body mechanics while working the arms during a Swedish massage. I am leaning back and giving the client a spinal twist/stretch using their arm. I am not lifting her up or using extraneous muscle to perform the task. Instead, I am leaning back and almost falling back but holding on to her arm to prevent me from falling back.

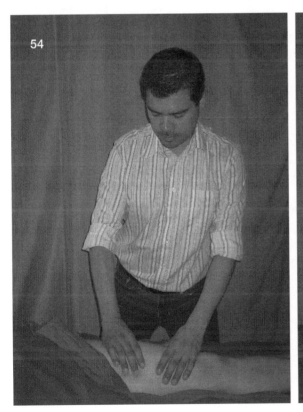

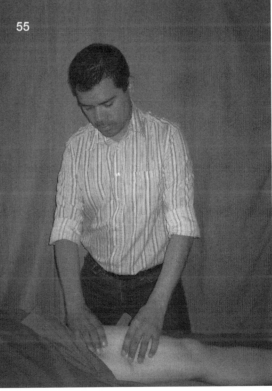

Photos 54 & 55: As I petrissage the quadriceps, as with other petrissages, my whole body moves side to side, not just my hands. Although some petrissage strokes are taught as gripping strokes, notice I am not gripping or grasping with my hands. Instead, the motion of my body allows my hands to move side to side. My chest is open, allowing me to easily take in air and move freely. Notice my elbows are not out but instead, close to my body. Finally, I am focused on the work yet my head is not dropped.

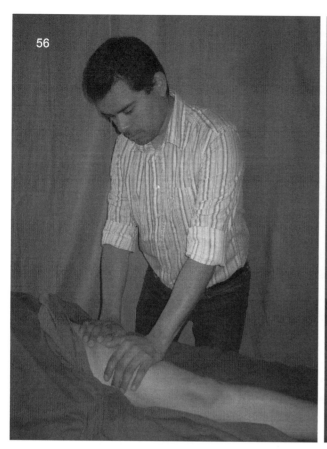 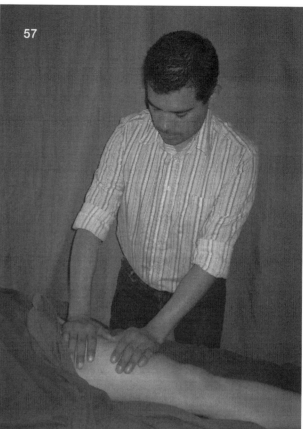

Photos 56 and 57: In working in a cross fiber manner on the quadriceps muscles, my hands are showing the end result of my hips and the rest of my body rotating in a clock-wise then counter clock-wise manner. In Photo 56 my left hip is going forward as my left hand moves forward. In photo 57, my right hip moves forward as my right hand moves forward. Notice my shoulders are stable and not going up to perform the movement. Using my whole body and not just the areas that most of us usually rely on means I have more energy to work the rest of the day.

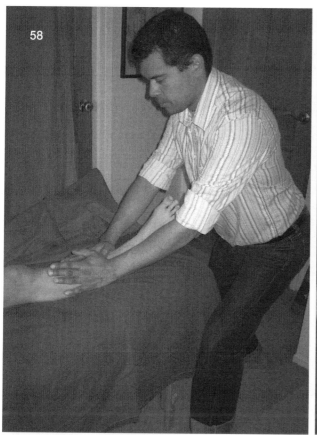

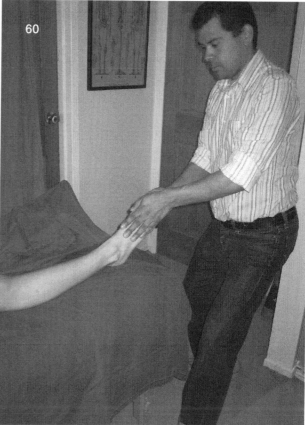

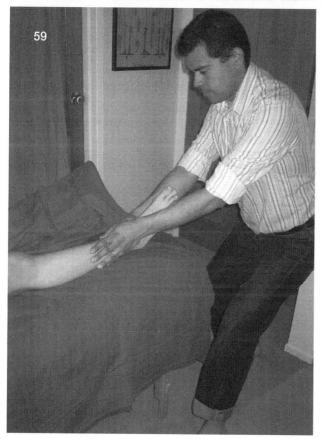

Photos 58, 59, and 60: In doing an effleurage on the lower leg, again my whole body moves forward in a sort of lunge movement. My hands are out and the force that is created by this movement is transferred in the form of a stroke onto the client's lower leg. As I lean forward most of the weight is on my left leg and as I lean back to complete the stroke, the weight is mainly transferred to my back leg. Remember however the movement is not just coming from the legs but from the whole body. Finishing the stroke can be accomplished at the feet where by then I would be standing up a bit more and able to lean forward and backward at a slow rhythmic pace and using that movement to work the feet.

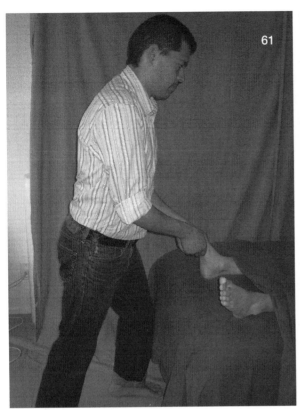

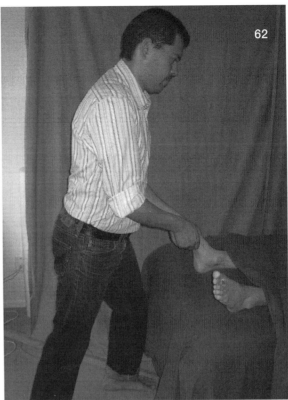

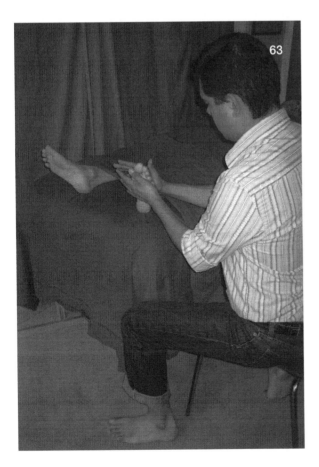

Photos 61 and 62 (ABOVE): Working the feet is also possible in this forward stance. Here I am using my hands to work the feet without having to muscle it. I have my forefingers on the sole of the foot while my thumbs are on the dorsal part. As I lean forward, having this hold bends the foot and brings my forefingers deeper into the foot. As I lean back, holding on to the foot creates a slight stretch. All this is done without having to over-grip the foot at all but instead use kinetic energy and the power of leverage. This same movement can also be used to create a slight tug on each toe, one at a time. When I slightly tug on each toe, I am mindful that it is not just my hands that are working on the client's foot but my whole body. If you work this way you will notice that not only is the client's foot moving, but their whole body is being moved by this way of working.

Photo 63 (LEFT): Even in sitting I can use my whole body to create a stroke on the feet. Here I am rocking on my ischial tuberosities while I am also working the feet with my hands in a sort of 'sandwich' way. The movement of my body creates ease in the movement of my hands. Notice my back is still pretty straight and my hands are relatively relaxed. The table height is also at a level that is comfortable for me. If the table was a bit high I would have stood up and bent my knees (in Forward Stance) to a comfortable level for my whole body.

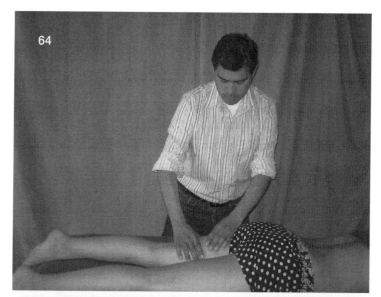

Photos 64 and 65: In performing a petrissage on the hamstrings, the same side to side movement is employed. Although my elbows are out, the movement of my body going side to side is what is creating the stroke. Notice in the photo you can tell when my right hand is primarily working the hamstrings, my left knee is bent (again, creating the movement towards the left and forcing the right hand to move left). When my left hand is primarily working, my right knee is bent, forcing my body to move to the right and my left hand to move to the right.

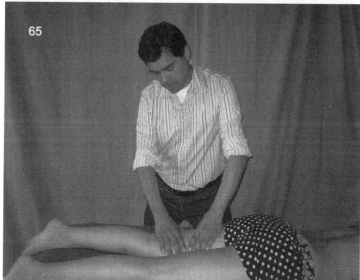

The main point behind the photos and their captions is to emphasize and illustrate the main principle of Swedish massage body mechanics. In all of those photos I meant to show that proper movement is necessary to create the strokes. Again, I don't recommend you aim to mimic the strokes exactly. Instead, understand the principles and allow your strokes to take their own unique form using the photos as a template.

CHAPTER 7:

THE BEGINNINGS OF DEEP TISSUE BODY MECHANICS

Introduction

There is a distinct difference between body mechanics for Swedish massage and Deep Tissue massage. In Swedish, we aim to create movement in our bodies that will ultimately translate into movement of our hands, forearms or soft fist. This works great when we are attempting to move along more or less the transverse plane and move more superficial tissue. When we are aiming to work a deeper layer of tissue, we need to access it. One way would be to use brute force to force our way into that deeper layer. The other way would be to exploit gravity and let our selected tool be an extension of our bodies as we employ the mass of our bodies to create a force that will be used to sink into the deeper layer of tissue. This is also in conjunction and in concert (speed is key here) with the tissue's reaction to the mass of the practitioner. The latter form of usage of the body is more economical and allows the practitioner to avoid injury while also avoiding an injury to the client.

Body awareness exercises for Deep Tissue Body Mechanics

As with Swedish massage there are a couple of body awareness exercises that I share with my students before we venture into deep tissue territory. These exercises help to explain how to use our bodies in a more efficient manner without strain.

The Bicep Load exercise

This exercise was taught to me during my Rolfing training. A willing student is asked to lift up his hand, palm up, bending the elbow at a 90 degree angle. I place a light object on his hand (a pen for example) and he is asked if he can feel the weight of the object on his palm. The student will usually say that he can barely feel it but that he does feel it. Next, the pen is taken away and a load is placed on the hand. I usually put a few books on it, just enough for him to start employing his bicep muscle while still keeping his elbow bent at 90 degrees. Once I see that he is doing that, I then place the pen on top of the books and ask him the same question, "Can you feel the weight of the pen?" The student will then say that he can no longer feel the weight of the pen.

What ends up happening here is that there is so much of a load being placed on the biceps due to the books that the student will lose sense of the smallest increment in weight or pressure. If he can not feel the pen, how can he expect to feel what may be happening to the client's muscle/connective tissue under their hands/fist/elbow if he is overusing his muscles? This exercise has helped me throughout my bodywork career and allows me to relax and sink deeper into the work. Having your muscles overly contracted may also cause the client to tense up by the mere fact that they are feeling the practitioner's muscle contractions. One massage therapy instructor describes this possibility as the "telegraphing of strain."

The Lean (employing the ankle joints)

A lot of us may not be using our whole entire body when doing deep tissue work. In fact, using just a bit more of your whole self may be all that's necessary in order to do more effective and efficient work. The following exercise was shown to me by a deep tissue instructor who I incorrectly assumed would not have enough mass or strength to do deeper work. I was completely mistaken when she used me as a demonstration model! The following is a breakdown of the exercise as I have modified it and shown it. I first have a student stand in front of me and we are both facing each other, both with our feet hip width apart. I then ask the student to put their hand out and place their palm on my chest, in effect not allowing me to move forward if I wanted to. I then attempt to move forward without moving my feet. First I lean head first, as if I'm moving forward from my head. After that doesn't work, I bend at my hip, still attempting to move forward. In both cases the student is easily able to resist my moving forward. The reason is because I am not employing my whole self in the process. An important step in the 'whole self' process is leaning

forward from the ankles. The more stuck we get in a habitual pattern the more we attempt to walk and move in all sorts of different ways and we discard the potential of our ankles. Take a look at people walking along a busy street and you'll notice lack of movement in the ankles from a lot of them. They will use/overuse other parts of their bodies to propel themselves forward and end up shuffling or hobbling along. So, in my final attempt I keep my body straight, employ my ankles and lean forward using my ankles as a hinge. Invariably the student needs to take a step back and get into a lunge position in order to resist me moving forward. From here the exercise could take on more of an exercise in movement awareness if I move forward employing my bent ankles while the student gives me minor resistance. Photo 66 shows an illustration of the lean. Notice how I am keeping one foot back to prevent from falling backward and that the model is looking in the direction where she's leaning. Essentially, she's looking where she's going! If you have issues or limitations in your ankles, do this exercise to bring more movement to the ankles.

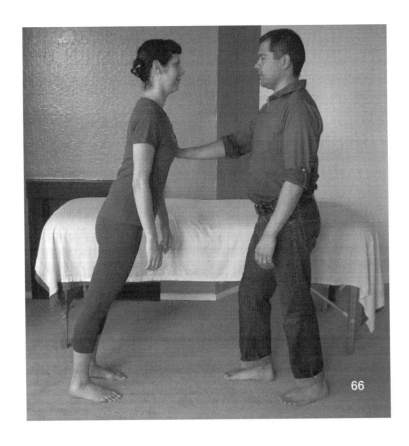
66

Transversus Abdominis

I was originally taught to imagine my strokes coming from my core. As I have been working throughout these years, I now believe the 'core' is a great way to begin in body mechanics but is not the main source of the strokes. Instead, as I have said before, the whole self needs to be employed to create the work. This means that the core also needs to be employed in addition to everything else. When I take my students through the core engagement process, I emphasize the transversus abdominis. An easy way to engage this muscle is to bring the belly button slightly towards the spinal column. It doesn't need to be a full-on workout, just enough to engage the core while employing the whole body. Engaging the transversus abdominis while employing the ankles helps to stabilize the low back during deep tissue work.

Gravity is the Principle, Economy is the Technique

Before I move on to teach my students the physical aspects of body mechanics and share with them the way I work in Deep Tissue, I share the two simple things they need to remember to employ proper body mechanics. GRAVITY IS THE PRINCIPAL. It's as easy as that. Gravity is your friend and can be exploited for the cause. As I teach techniques, I tell my students to not attempt to memorize them or worse yet, to mimic me. Instead, I tell them to remember the other rule: Economy is the technique. ECONOMY IS THE TECHNIQUE. I tell my students to not strive to mimic me because we all have different body structures and come to the table with different ways of using our bodies. The client's proportions and the table height also change how we work. Therefore, our techniques are derived from understanding we can exploit gravity and find the most economical way to work. Understanding this also allows for more freedom in variation of techniques.

The Deep Tissue 'Jab'

In performing any deeper tissue technique with knuckles or soft fist I have noticed that less strain occurs up at the shoulder joint, elbow joint, and the wrist joint when the hand that is performing the technique is supported by its corresponding leg. For example, if I was going to do a deep tissue stroke on someone's hamstring with my left soft fist then my left leg would be in front, working in the human stance. I have found that this is very efficient and uses less energy than having the right leg forward. It also minimizes the twisting of the torso and makes for a deeper stroke. I equate this stroke to a slow motion version of a boxer's jab.

Do we need to 'push off'?

For massage, which does not require an explosive strike, pushing off with the back foot is not necessary. Some deep tissue instructors will show their techniques and encourage to push off from the back foot. This is a great way of doing the work but in the case of the way I'm teaching, when I'm doing deep tissue work I don't need to push off from my back foot because the leaning of my body and the fact that I'm using my whole self means that the force is being created by my body weight and not by muscular action such as pushing off. Instead of pushing off, I suggest employing the ankles and exploiting gravity to dissipate any stress response and allow the practitioner to use their whole body weight to lean into the client's tissue, creating a deep tissue stroke that way.

CHAPTER 8:

BODY MECHANICS FOR DEEP TISSUE MASSAGE

The following is a set of photos showing some deep tissue strokes that use the principles previously described. One thing I want to point out is that you may notice that I am not leaning as much as shown in the 'Lean' exercise and I may be bending at the waist in addition to bending at the ankles. If properly employed, leaning at the ankles creates tremendous force since you're using your whole body. You will in fact notice that you don't need to lean as much to sink into deeper layers of tissue ("I don't have to work as hard!" you might say) or it may feel like you're barely working (based on our previously held notions of what work might be). You might notice you will have to hold back a bit so you don't injure the client by sinking in too deep too fast or working too fast. In my work I can say that I rarely use even 90% of my effort in performing deeper work such as Rolfing® or Deep Tissue Massage. Usually my effort (when I employ proper body mechanics) hovers around 30-40% and that is enough to do great work. An important thing to note is that I have been using these techniques for years and I am aware that it may take a while for bodyworkers to get used to using new techniques. Tendons and ligaments need to strengthen and different muscles are used when new techniques are employed.

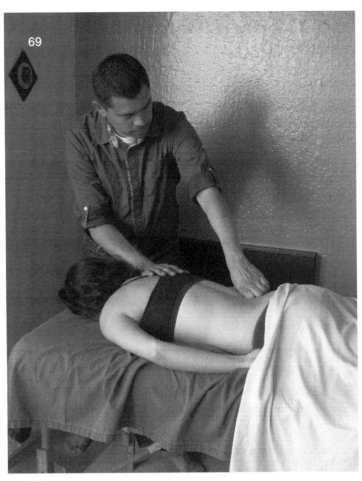

Photo 69: In working the back, I am showing how two knuckles can be employed to work the lower back muscles. I am slowing leaning into the tissue and my other hand is resting on the client, supporting me and giving the client a sense of connection. The main thing to notice here is my wrist. Notice it is not curved or tweaked, instead it is fairly straight. My left shoulder is also not any higher than my right shoulder. All the force of my lean is going into my client's low back. And since I don't need to fully lean to sink deep into the tissue, the lean is not extremely pronounced. In this case, my left leg is forward as is my left arm.

Photo 70: The same technique can be used from the other direction to work the lower back going in the direction of the client's head. In this case my left hand is on my client's right foot and my right soft fist is working up the erectors. My left hand doesn't have much weight resting on it (my wrist is relaxed) and most my weight is resting on the right soft fist. Having my hands in this position allows me to be supported while doing the work. Notice my shoulders are still relaxed and the right wrist is still straight.

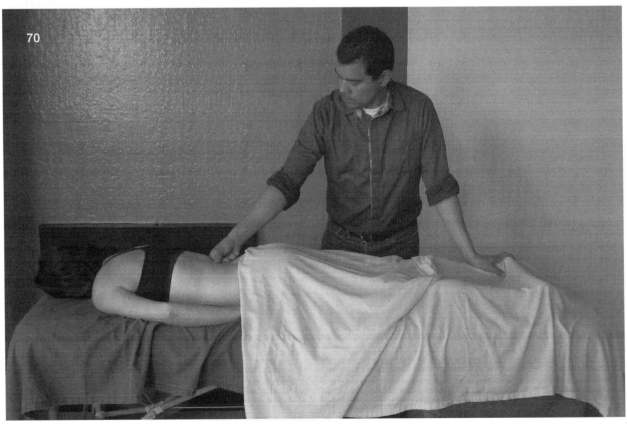

Photo 71: In this photo I am working along the erectors. I am using my whole forearm, not just my elbow. I am sitting on the table and my client's arm is bent over my left leg which is on the table also. This allows me to sit on the table and lean into my client's back tissue, letting my full upper body become the tool instead of just my arm. Notice also my left wrist is relaxed, not tense. I am mindful not to go directly on the spinous process of course. This stroke is very effective and can deliver great access to a deeper layer of tissue depending on the lean of my upper body. This stroke is also very effective when working in small, cramped spaces where a bodyworker may not have the space to move around the table.

Photos 72 and 72b: This back stroke is very effective and not only aims at working deep tissue of the back but also specifically aims to work the fascial layer underneath the erectors. My right leg is forward (still in the forward stance) and my right forearm is acting like a 'blade' and I'm imagining slicing underneath the layer of the erectors. I jokingly call this stroke 'filleting' as you can imagine the movement of the ulna on the back is similar to the filleting of a fish. This stroke actually accesses the layer of fascia under the erectors, a layer of fascia that is often ignored in a deep tissue back massage. My whole body is behind the tool (in this case the 'blade') as I'm bending from the ankles and leaning in to perform the work. Photo 72b shows the stroke from a different angle. In both photos, notice my head is up and not dropped.

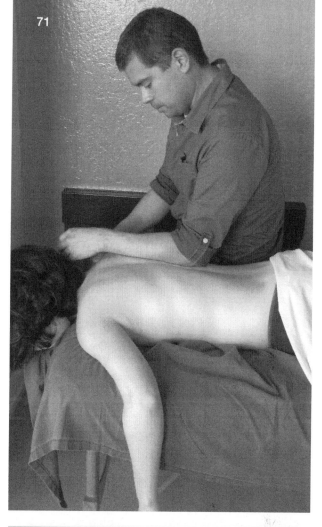

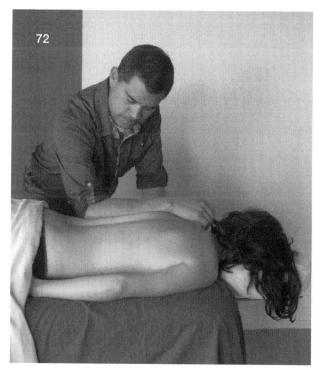

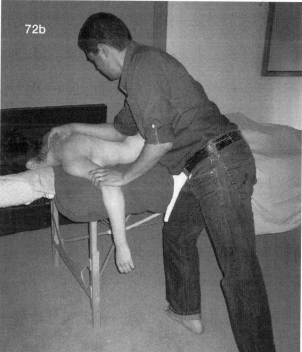

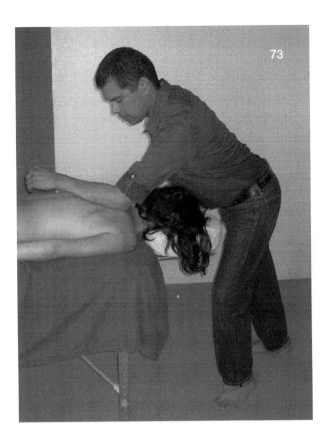

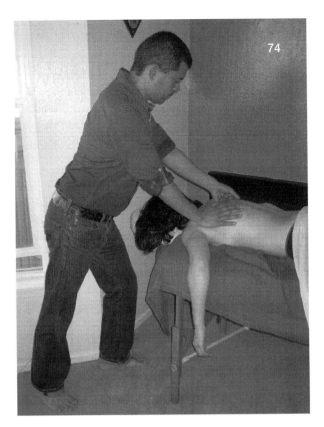

Photo 73: The lower part of my forearm is the tool that is translating my gravity into work in this stroke. I am leaning forward with my whole body and I'm sinking into the muscle tissue attached to the medial border of the scapula. As previously noted, I am relaxed and allowing my whole mass to be the force behind this work. I am coming at this tissue not head on but from an angle so as not bump up with the client's head. Again, I am barely using any strength and if I am, it's actually to hold back from sinking in too fast and causing the client pain. Notice my left foot is supporting my left forearm/elbow by being the forward foot.

Photo 74: Here's an example of working the same area but in a confined space. I know that some massage therapists for all sorts of reasons end up working in small rooms. If there is no space to do the previous move, then move off to one side, stack the joints, and bend those ankles as you're using your soft fist. If you're finding yourself raising your shoulders then maybe the table is too high. If so, and you can't easily lower the table, then it might be time to do the stroke in Photo 71 as that stroke will level the playing field so to speak when it comes to table height. Notice my back is relatively straight and my left wrist is not tweaked or twisted. This stroke has a 'short commute' as I call it, meaning I don't go down the whole back with this stroke. If I did, then my wrist would bend and my bones would not stack. For this reason, the distance this stroke can travel is limited.

A Note on Hyper-Flexibility

You may have seen in the previous photo my bones are stacked and my arm is straight at the elbow. You may have seen this photo and have thought, "That's great that he can do that but when I try my elbow hyper-extends and my wrists don't seem to want to stack!" I have seen plenty of students and bodyworkers that have hyper-mobile or hyper-flexible joints and to them I say to experiment with stacking bones and see how that feels. Inevitably students will tell me that their arm or wrists feels bent (flexed) but yet to look at it, it is stacked. Working this way may feel different, or even odd. Muscles and tendons are not used to stopping at that point and may feel sore after working like this for a bit. If working this way doesn't feel comfortable at all, don't worry. As a teacher once told me, "There are a billion strokes out there". When I work with students who are hyper-mobile, I spend some time to find out what the best way of working is for them and how can they use their body more efficiently, effectively, and safely.

Photo 75: In this photo I am working on the upper trapezius muscles in a sitting position. I believe this is one of the most efficient ways to work this tissue when the client is prone. Being in the sitting position gives me the opportunity to approach the tissue directly and along the same plane. Notice my wrist is relaxed and I'm near the edge of the chair. This allows me to lean forward more and easily apply more force. As an added bonus, my left hand is by the client's occipital area. What I'm doing there is providing an anchor point in order to increase the effectiveness of what's happening under my right forearm. I'm not muscling with my left hand, just gently creating an anchor point so my left wrist is not strained.

Photos 76 and 76b: Another variation of working the same upper trapezius tissue is to use knuckles. Notice I've straightened out my arm and have turned my palm away from the camera. This allows for better aligning of the bones and joints in the hand and therefore better transmission of force through the arm. Because I'm using my whole arm now I need to sit back in the chair to allow for the added distance. I am also reaching closer to the occiput with my other hand, increasing the lengthening of the tissue. This working with both hands allows for more work to occur without me having to work as 'hard'. "Twice the work for half the effort" is what I tell my students. Photo 76b shows a better view of what is happening under the knuckles. Notice my hand in this photo has moved away from the client's left occipital area in order for the photo to show my right hand.

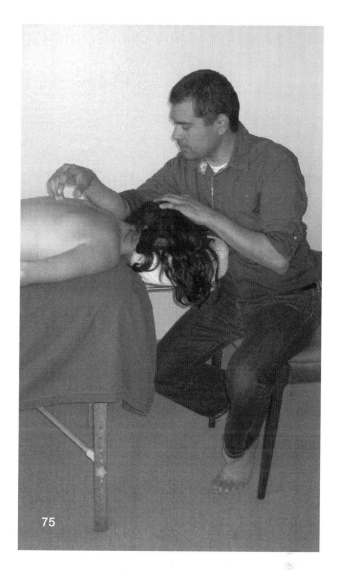

75

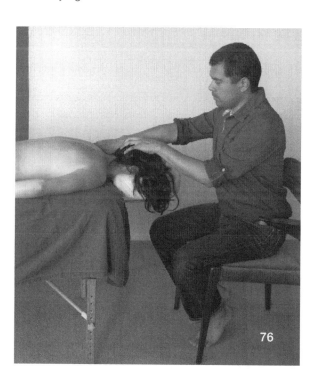

76

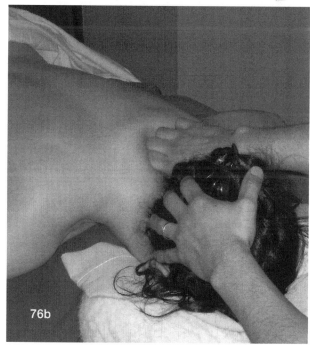

76b

Photo 77: Working the gluteal muscles in this manner allows me to use a good amount of my mass. My left forearm is at the perimeter of the ilium and my right forearm is close to the scapula. Now comes the easy part, I lean! I'm mindful of where my forearms are and I can shift my weight to either forearm. Notice that my right foot is slightly more forward than the left foot. I'm still in a Forward Stance which prevents me from inadvertently using my low back to straighten up; instead I can use my front foot to stand up by pushing back with my front foot then bend the back leg. Another way out of this stroke is to bend my back leg as if I'm about to kneel then stand up using my front leg muscles. This method allows me to bring my pelvic girdle underneath my head and not use my back muscles to straighten up.

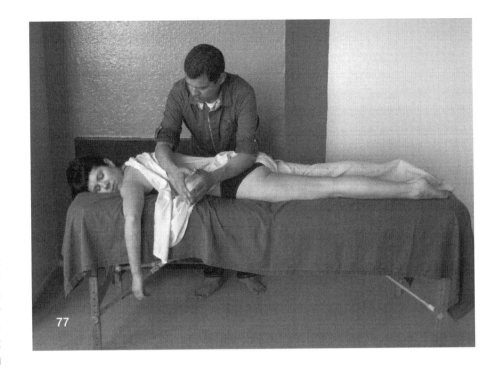

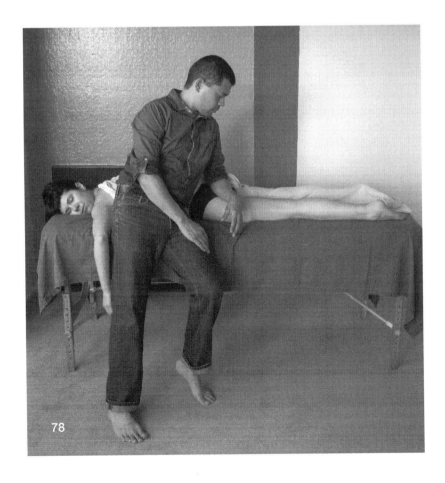

Photo 78: I have found this deep tissue stroke very helpful in working the quadratus femoris muscle. I am using a bit of the table to lean on and my elbow and forearm are resting right on the area of the quadratus femoris. Notice the relaxed posture. I am focused on the work and also focused on my left shoulder. The shoulder is not raised and I am monitoring if there is any strain there. I don't want my shoulder to be too far away from my body. I am not moving with this stroke (I sometimes see massage therapists use this technique but then move their forearm towards themselves in order to work the tissue, a big no-no) as that would put more strain on the shoulder girdle muscle and lead to possible overuse/strain. Instead, I'm waiting for the tissue to allow me to sink into it more then I might move slightly but not a lot. Again, if I have space limitations, I may go to this stroke.

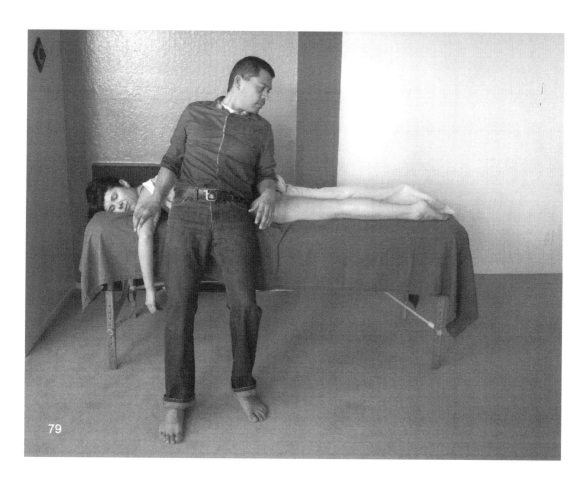

79

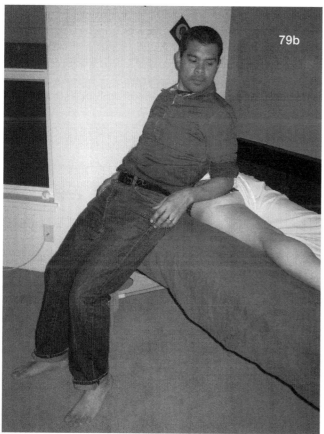

79b

Photos 79 and 79b: If I am dealing with a particularly tight set of gluteal muscles or with an individual much larger than myself then I might employ a technique I learned in Brazil in order to get more of my mass behind the tool. In this case I am fully leaning on the table and my left forearm has more of my upper body behind it compared to the previous technique. Of course, I am still waiting to sink into the tissue and not forcing the tissue to do anything it doesn't want to do. Even though I am leaning on the table I am careful not to have my body contact the client too much as I don't want to give the client the feeling that I'm resting on them. Photo 79b shows the technique from a different angle. I have been mentioning before about how my hand is relaxed or my shoulder is relaxed but in Photo 79b you can definitely see how my face and feet are also relaxed. Being focused on the work entails focus that is not derived by intensity but rather a focus that flows from a place of relaxation. I am reminded of Monica Caspari, a Rolf Movement teacher who taught me to assess clients with 'soft eyes'.

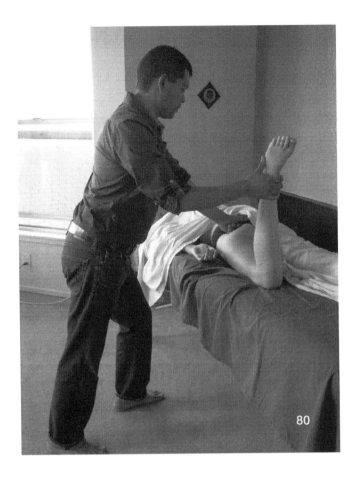

80

Photo 80: The body mechanics in this photo are similar to many others but I like to show this technique because it illustrates a method that Art Riggs, Certified Advanced Rolfer™ calles 'anchor and stretch'. My left soft fist anchors in the muscle tissue (in this case the piriformis) while my right hand stretches the leg by moving the client's foot towards the left (in this photo in the direction where I'm at but not necessarily towards me). This in effect stretches the piriformis tissue under my soft fist. I like to show this photo because it's easy to combine this technique with the one in Photo 79 to create one 'super technique'. In that technique I would lean on the client as I am in Photo 79 while I ask the client to raise their foot (bending at the knee) and move their foot towards the left hand side of the table. Again, I employ minimal (yet focused) effort but achieve maximum results. As before, my wrists is not bent or angled, all my bones are aligned.

Photo 81: Here you see me working the gluteal muscles from another direction. I'm still using the table as a support and controlling my leaning to work the upper gluteal muscles. Although I'm on the table I'm not unnecessarily leaning or touching my client. This technique can be used to also work the sacrotuberus ligament. My wrist is relaxed and my feet/toes are relaxed. My elbow is not too far away from my body (doing so would put undue strain on my shoulder girdle). Being able to fully relax allows me to focus more on the work and be present with the client. Even though I'm not leaning with my whole body there is enough mass in the upper body to create the force necessary to slowly sink into the tissue. Notice my left foot is not close to the table instead is creating a support so I keep my balance without strain.

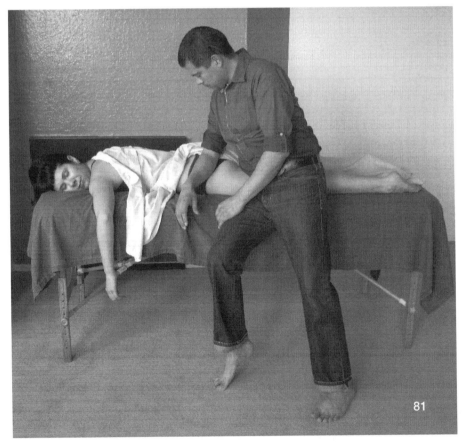

81

A Break for Physics

There are some brilliant massage teachers out there. Some have employed Newtonian laws to describe what is necessary in order to perform deep tissue work. I have seen and been taught the law of

$$F=ma$$

as it is used to explain deep tissue work where F equals Force, m equals mass and a equals acceleration (in its most basic and simple sense). I have come to learn however that:

$$F=mg$$

is a better way of recognizing what happens during deep tissue work. F=ma is more often used to explain thrust in airplanes or automobiles. If we use it to explain the mechanics behind deep tissue work then we are required to come up with a source for the acceleration. In its best case, it will fall to the task of the back foot as I have explained before that some instructors will have their students use. In its worst case,

the task of coming up with acceleration will fall to our muscles where muscles will be used to propel ourselves forward and we are back where we started, using (and most likely overusing) muscle which will take us down a spiral path of possible injury.

Now, if we use F=mg where F equals Force, m equals mass and g equals gravity, we have the makings for a slightly different philosophy for deep tissue work. Instead of having to come up with a method of acceleration, we can instead use gravity (which incidentally, is a unit of acceleration). Of course, I understand that some muscle is necessary to bring body off balance but it's not anymore muscle action than is necessary to maintain the act of standing up straight. As I have said before, we should exploit gravity in order to create this work. F=mg is used more to measure falling objects. So, what if we saw ourselves as 'falling' onto the tissue in a controlled manner and with attention to 'falling' on a specific location? We now have physics on our side to support the previous statement of "Gravity is the principle".

Photo 82: In this technique, my forefinger and my middle finger knuckle are the end points for my force, The joints are stacked and the muscles and tendons of the wrists and arm don't need to work as much as a result.

This photo reveals a good amount with respect to my body mechanics. There is a lean here in my pelvic girdle. This however is not the only place where the lean is being generated. Notice the bend in my right ankle. I am leaning forward using my ankles as a hinge. This allows more of my mass to get behind the stroke. As you can tell, I don't need to lean that much in order to go into a deeper layer of tissue. My right hand is supporting me in this endeavor and I 'close the circuit' by resting it on my client's foot. This technique works the Peroneal muscles very well.

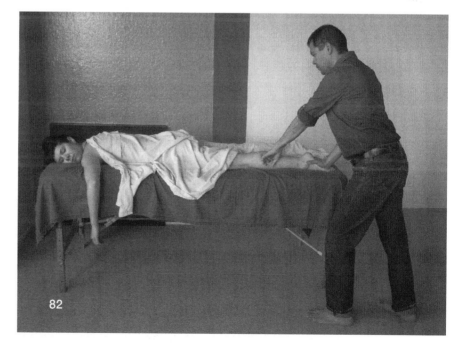

82

Photo 83: Still working on the lower leg, I have adjusted my body to be able to work the medial muscles of the lower leg (Tibialis Posterior, for example). Notice that I raised my right leg and put my right knee on the table. I also moved to the other side of the table. When showing this to my students, I equate this to billiards. My right arm is straight like a cue stick and I am looking for the best angle to bring my tool (in this case two knuckles at the end of a straight arm) to the tissue. Since my right leg is off the floor, I will be using my hip as the hinge. I will be leaning slightly forward from my hip, keeping my back straight. The straightness of my right arm makes it easy for the force to easily translate into the client's lower leg. I am still using the premise of keeping my lead foot (or in this case leg) forward even though it's off the table. My left leg acts a balance for the rest of my body.

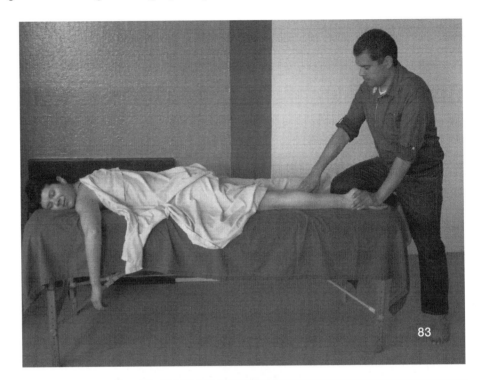

Photo 84: Using the same billiards analogy, I can find the right geometry/angle to employ my straightened arm to work the medial hamstrings. Notice I put my knee up slightly on the table. This is meant to give me a bit more height in order to approach the hamstring tissue from the most efficient angle. If I were to use an electric table, I would lower it slightly in order to get a better angle and I wouldn't need to get on the table. If the circumstances don't allow for that, then I find the best angle by slightly getting on the table. Again, be mindful of not leaning on your client or sending the wrong signal.

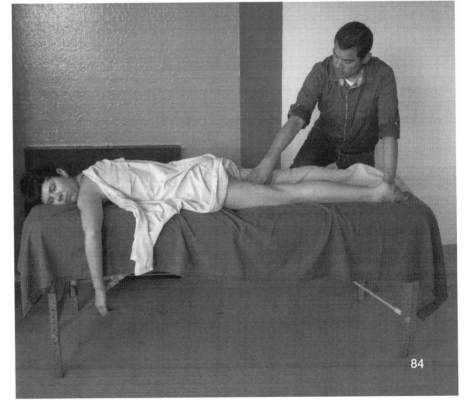

Photos 85 and 86: Notice when I move to the other side of the table and don't get on the table, I don't have the height to be able to work on the top part of the hamstrings. In Photo 85 my forearm muscles are visibly engaging. I have to use more muscle and I will most likely be fighting a losing battle with the client's hamstrings using this technique. Instead, I can use more of my upper body weight, lean on the table, and use my forearm to work the hamstrings. If I want to pinpoint some tissue or a fascial septum, I can raise my hand up so my elbow is more pointed and able to sink into the tissue as a point and not as a blunt tool like the forearm. This technique may look different than the way you may have been taught: no legs on the table, left leg forward and moving forward along the hamstrings with your right forearm. Although a fantastic technique, I don't use that method since it uses more muscle and energy (not as efficient) as the technique in photo 86.

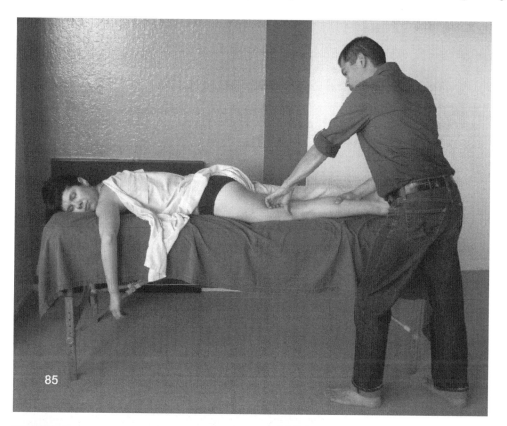

85

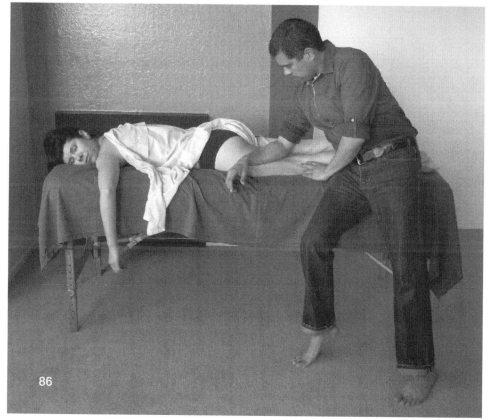

86

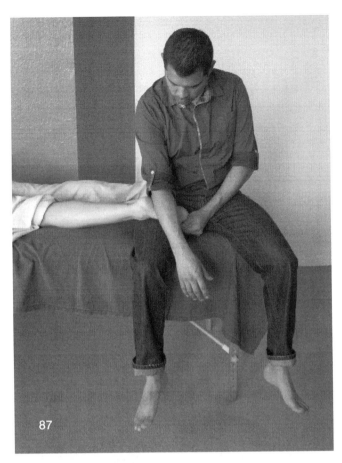

87

Photos 87, 88 and 88b: Using the blunt part or the pointy part of the elbow can come in handy when working on the feet. Notice I'm not using thumbs or fingers to work the feet when the client is in prone position. Instead, I sit on the table and have the clients' foot over my leg. My left hand holds the foot in order to make sure the foot is not up near my inner thigh. My right elbow can easily work the heel or either of the arches by simply leaning into the foot. Any force created comes from my leaning into the foot and not from muscling it. As shown in Photo 88, I can apply more pinpoint pressure by raising my hand and creating a bony point to the elbow. If it seems like you might have to flex your torso too much in order to achieve this move, then you can simply cross your leg (in this case, the right leg over the left) or put a pillow under the foot. Either scenario will put the foot closer to the elbow and prevent any flexion or tweaks in your posture. Photo 88b shows an easy warm-up of the foot tissue. Notice I am not using my thumbs at all. I rarely use my thumbs when working the feet, but instead will use knuckles (in supine position) or elbows as seen in the earlier photos.

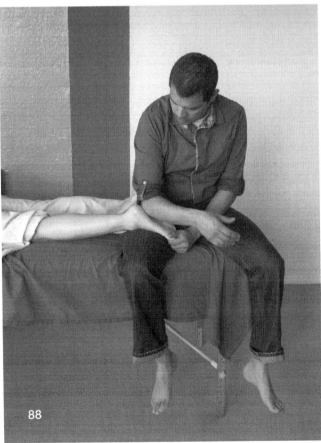

88

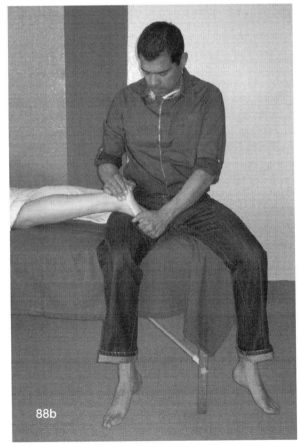

88b

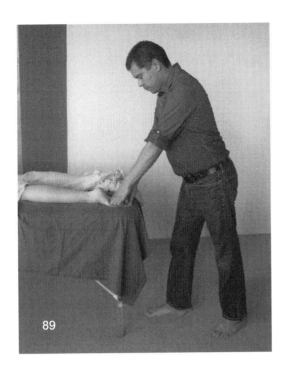

89

Photo 89: Keeping the same theme of working the feet, another way is to keep the client in prone and use either a soft fist or knuckles down the plantar fascia. Again, I don't have to lean in as much in order to get into the deeper layer of tissue on the foot. If I have a client with a lot of tissue in this area then I could lean into it some more, from the ankle joints, in order to get my whole body into stroke. Again, there only needs to be a slight leaning into the tissue that when it's seen in a photo, it may seem like I'm not leaning in at all. Experience this with a practicum to realize the power behind the lean. Also, be mindful of not dropping your head too much.

Photo 89: Keeping the same theme of working the feet, another way is to keep the client in prone and use either a soft fist or knuckles down the plantar fascia. Again, I don't have to lean in as much in order to get into the deeper layer of tissue on the foot. If I have a client with a lot of tissue in this area then I could lean into it some more, from the ankle joints, in order to get my whole body into stroke. Again, there only needs to be a slight leaning into the tissue that when it's seen in a photo, it may seem like I'm not leaning in at all. Experience this with a practicum to realize the power behind the lean. Also, be mindful of not dropping your head too much.

Photos 90 and 91: I've seen that for most folks, working the quadriceps muscles with a soft fist is sufficient. I can easily lean into it, feeling the hinge of my right ankle joint. Keeping my left arm straight in this photo again allows me to smoothly transfer my force into my client's quadriceps. If I need to work the area where the quadriceps make way to thicker connective tissue (aka IT band), then I can medially rotate the leg to expose the area I want to work on instead of having to twist my body to conform to the client's leg. But what if I wanted to work more on the medial part of the quadriceps? Instead of bending my arm at the elbow to conform to the shape of the leg, or worse, using my other arm to work the medial part, I will use a different tool. In Photo 91 I decide to use my forearm and half-sit on the table. Notice this move is exactly like the move I used to work on the hamstrings in Photo 86. I can now maneuver my forearm without strain to work vastus medialis. If I want to work more on the adductors, I can slightly externally rotate the leg. I take care to make sure I'm not leaning on the client's leg and that they are comfortable in their draping. In Photo 91 my left hand is not applying any pressure, instead is acting as a guide for the leg, making sure it's optimally angled. My shoulders are still not raised and my right foot is slightly off the ground, indicating that maybe the table is a bit high for my height. I'm countering this

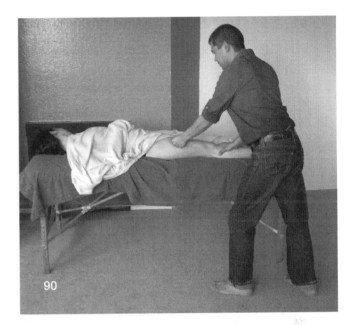

90

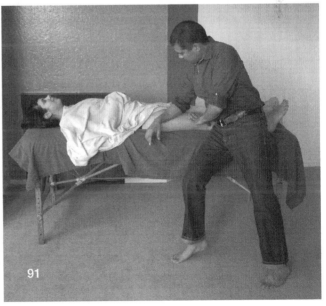

91

height by leaning on the table, putting myself slightly off balance to my right and as a result, the client's leg is taking on the force created by that off balance. If the table height was lower, then my foot would be flatter on the ground.

Sinking Into Tissue and Body Mechanics

My mentor has often told the story of when he was teaching a class to a group of very serious students. After a demonstration, one student asked him to explain how much pressure per square inch, how much duration in seconds, and how much travel in millimeters he was applying to the tissue. My mentor looked at him and gave him precise numbers for all requests! Of course, the answers were meant to be humorous. It's nearly impossible to create a precise formula that will tell how deeply to go into the tissue for how long; nevertheless, it is extremely important to know how to do this properly. Working too fast or applying too much pressure too quickly will almost always result in the client's tissue tensing up against the pressure. This of course is not conducive to good bodywork. Proper body mechanics aids in properly sinking into deeper layers of tissue. When a practitioner is using their body well, they will be aware of the proper amount of pressure to allow to happen and how much they need to sink into the tissue for that particular client at that particular point in time. What I see in beginning students is the tentativeness to sink into the tissue. They may sink into the tissue slightly then 'bounce' out. This bouncing in and out does not make for good work. Adopting a protocol of sinking then moving while you are using your body (incorporating the ankles) to lean into the tissue at the appropriate pace makes for much more effective, efficient, and safe work. What is the appropriate pace? This is where listening to the client is key. Listening not only to what they have to say but what their body may be telling you will create an action plan for the proper amount of pressure and travel when working deeply. This will then make for memorable work that will keep clients coming back.

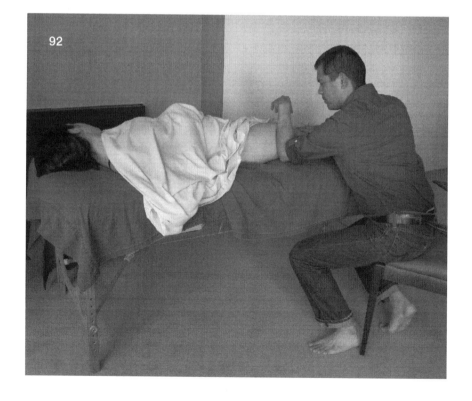

Photo 92: When teaching a body mechanics class I often see bodyworkers bring their elbow to their body and use their fist to work the IT band. This is a fine way to work this area but I make it a point to show them the following technique so they have more options to pull from. In this move, I am sitting down by the edge of the chair. Instead of a straight arm where the soft fist or knuckles or fingers are the end of the tool, the forearm is the end of the tool. Sitting at the edge of the chair allows me to be off balance enough so that the client's IT band is the recipient of the force created by my off balance. My right hand is also guiding the client's leg into medial rotation. This allows me to access more of the IT band. This is a 'short commute' technique, meaning I don't keep my lower body stationery while my left forearm moves up the IT band. This would put undo pressure in my rotator cuff area. Instead, I work a small amount of IT band then reposition myself to work higher up on the leg. Notice my left wrist is relaxed and not carrying any tension into the stroke.

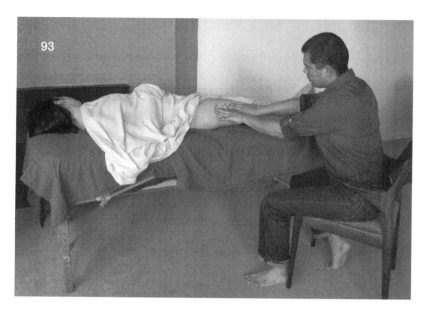

Photo 93: Another variation of the technique is to use fingers as a way to separate the compartments between Vastus Lateralis and IT band. Notice in this case I am further back in my chair. Because I'm using my fingers instead of forearm, I am able to put more pressure or force on a smaller surface area. This increases the level of intensity in the area without having to 'muscle' it at all. Specificity is key in this instance, not the muscle I can employ in my shoulders or arms.

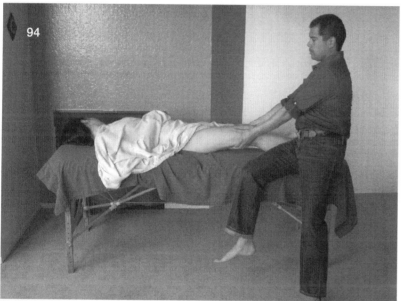

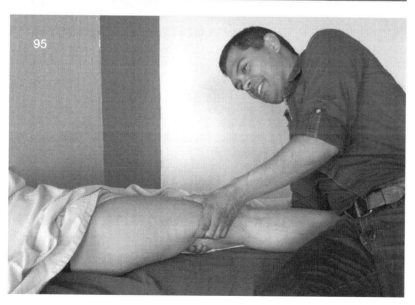

Photos 94 and 95: Sometimes you might remember you wanted to work the hamstrings when the client is in supine position but you may not know how to do it effectively. In Photo 94 I am reaching underneath the client's leg to work the compartments of the hamstring muscles. I am not grabbing or squeezing the tissue but instead I am using my body to make the stroke. I am leaning back and my client's leg is preventing me from falling backward. As I lean back my fingers slide toward the client's knee, working in between the fascial compartments. In Photo 95 I have medially rotated her leg only to show my hand placement, my left hand medial to the biceps femoris and my right hand medial to the semitendinosus muscle. It's important to note that when I'm sitting on the table, I take care to not have my pelvis rotated in one direction while my upper body is rotated in another direction. This is accomplished by having my right leg on the table, parallel to the client's leg. If this doesn't happen, then there may be too much torsion in my lower back.

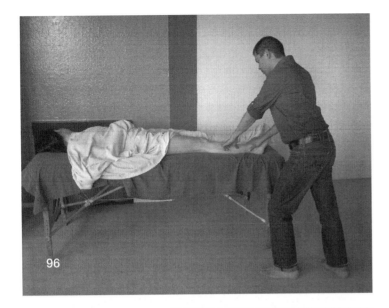

96

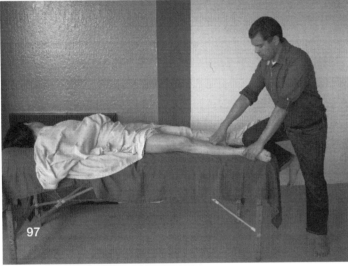

97

Photos 96 and 97: "One man's medicine is another man's poison". My mentor, Art Riggs, mentions this saying when speaking about techniques and bodywork approaches. I believe the same could be said to some extent regarding certain body mechanics and tools. As with the hamstrings in photos 83 and 84, I am using my knuckles to work the hamstring tissue. Again, the power comes from the lean. In teaching this stroke, I've found that bodyworkers who have not used their knuckles in this way do not have the strength to keep them straight and aligned. Because of this, I tell my students to try this technique but to also try using fingers, soft fists or forearms (as I did in photo 92) to work this area. Try different methods and see what works well for your body. Using the knuckles or fingers works really well for me but it may not necessarily be your thing. In Photo 96 I am clearly behind my tool (knuckles) as I lean in the tibialis anterior tissue. I am accessing the tissue better by medially rotating the leg with my right hand. In photo 97 I am using my knuckles to work the posterior compartment of the lower leg. Because this area requires specificity, I can also use fingers. As in photo 83, I am slightly on the table to allow me to raise my center of gravity up and then be able to bring it down on the lower leg via my knuckles. Notice I have also turned my client's leg out in order to access the tissue better. As with the other photos, I am not hunched over but instead keeping my back straight and leaning forward from my pelvis.

Photo 98: This technique, borrowed from Thai Massage, is a great example of using the whole body to perform a stroke. In this case I am on the table and have raised my client's leg and bent it at the knee. I have part of my right leg on her foot to stabilize the leg. My fingers are grabbing the tissue of the gastrocnemius much in the same way I was grabbing the hamstring tissue in Photo 94. Again, as I lean back I am exploiting gravity to create force on the gastrocnemius muscle. With a rhythmic motion, I can work all parts of this tissue systematically, moving up then down the posterior part of the lower leg. A variation of this work would be to use the rhythmic motion to not only work with gastrocnemius (and soleus) muscles with your fingers but also to lean forward and work the tibialis anterior muscles with the palm of the hand (in this case my left hand). Make sure your client is properly draped when doing this stroke.

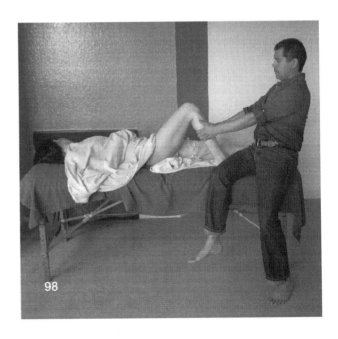

98

Photo 99: A great way to work the adductors deeply is to bring the leg out and use a forearm to sink into the tissue. The natural, relaxed position of my body allows me to sense how much to sink into the tissue and what pace I want to take. This work can also be accomplished in standing with a soft fist or in the same position as seen in the photo and using fingers. As you can tell in this photo, my left hand is stabilizing the client's leg but I am not muscling it to keep it stable. A note on draping: Notice the client's leg is draped snug. In this case I have wrapped the sheet around and under the client's leg. In my practice most of my clients are women and they have helped me learn how to be more considerate and properly

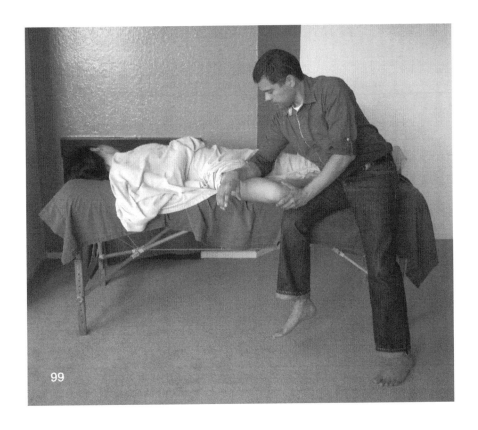

drape all my clients and use different tools that may make the work more comfortable for everyone. In this case I use my forearm. A forearm can seem less invasive for the client. If I use fingers, I usually work around the midpoint of the adductors. If I need to do any detail work on the upper part of the adductors, I will usually put the client in side lying position (more on that later).

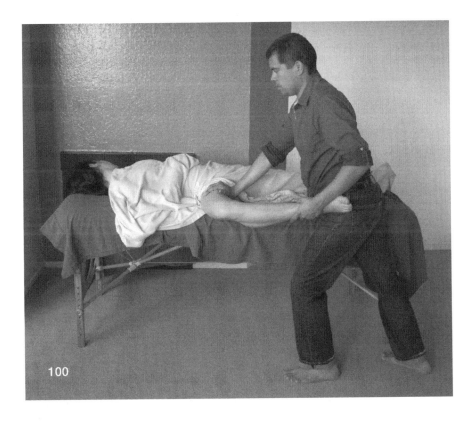

Photo 100: In this photo I am working the adductors with my right hand as my left hand stabilizes the leg. My left hand can either be on the client's foot or on the knee, depending which area gives the most stability. I steadily lunge forward and I lunge into the adductors. My arm is relatively straight, not bent (bending it would add strain to the shoulder) and the pressure is coming from the heel of my palm, not the center of it (where the carpal tunnel would be). It's important to note that I am able to comfortably do this stroke but if your wrists are sensitive and do not respond well to this move, then don't do it. Again, one man's medicine is another man's poison.

76

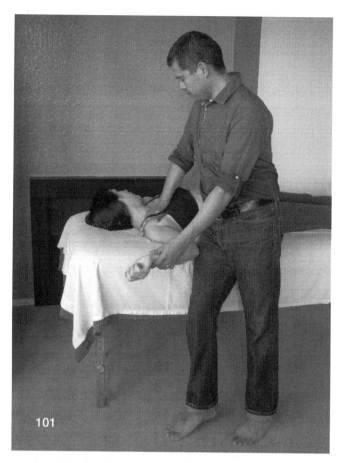

101

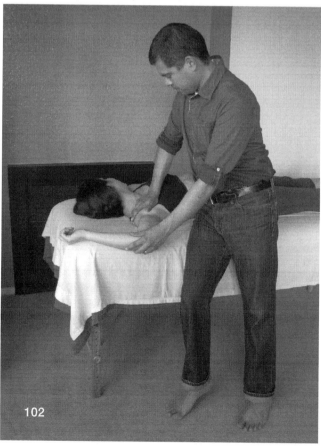

102

Photos 101 and 102: Doing deep tissue work on the pectoralis major muscle in this manner is simple and effective. In Photo 101 I am leaning on the table and my right hand is on the pectoral muscle, using the clavicle as a guide (without putting pressure on the clavicle). The area of my right hand that is applying pressure on the pectoral muscle is the thenar eminence (the fleshy part below my thumb) and not my carpal tunnel. My left hand is bringing the client's arm out. This stretches the pectoralis major muscle at the same time that I'm leaning on it. Notice that I am putting my right leg forward but if this causes undue torque on your spine, you can switch legs; essentially find the best fit for your body. In Photo 102, I am moving the client's arm from the elbow and instead of moving the arm out, I am moving the arm superiorly. This causes a stretch on the pectoralis minor versus the pectoralis muscle. Again, I'm leaning on the table a bit and using my upper body to work the tissue. Notice in Photo 102 my elbow is out a bit. At this point, I'm not applying a lot of pressure so having my elbow out might work in this instance. If I start to feel strain anywhere in my shoulder, I change strategies.

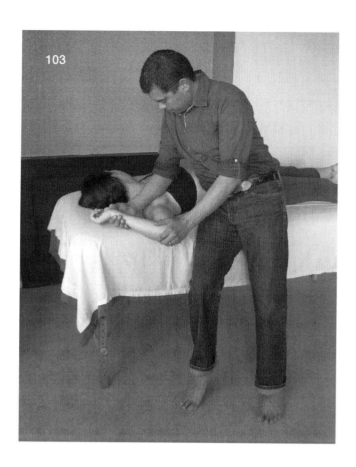

Photo 103: If I need to apply more pressure on the pectoralis tissue (let's say I'm working on a very muscular individual or can't seem to get the previous techniques to work for me) then I may opt to work it in this way. Here I am leaning more in the table and my forearm and elbow are on the pectoralis tissue. I am not using the pointy part of my elbow, rather the two or three inches of ulna before elbow. My right hand is holding the client's right hand and my left hand is holding her elbow. This allows me to move the arm down, out, or up, depending on which area of muscle tissue I want to work on. My right arm and shoulder is completely relaxed. The elbow makes a slow sweeping motion with about two to three inches of travel. The leaning in on the table allows me to put my weight more directly on top of the tissue I'm working and will prevent me from having to use my muscle to move across the tissue. Again, watch that the pelvis is not overly rotated. This technique creates a tremendous amount of pressure on the pectoralis muscle and requires focus and listening in order to prevent injuring the client.

Photo 104: If deep but specific work is necessary for the pecs and I need to use my fingers to get in between tissue, I will work from across the table. Instead of bending my knees and sinking from that way (as is usually taught and is a perfectly good way of working) I will opt to work with my right knee up on the table. This bring me closer to the client (of course be mindful not to put your knee too close to their face) and also puts me a bit off balance. This off balance is my exploitation of gravity that carries through my upper body into my fingers. I am then able to focus on finding the area I want to work on and any increase in pressure is a by-product of proper body

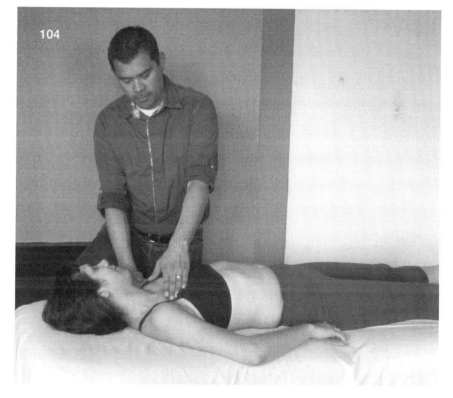

mechanics. Notice my arms are straight and shoulders are relaxed. If you feel that your client may not be comfortable with this way of working, then move on to something else. There are countless way of working and a vast majority of them will aid you to employ proper body mechanics.

Photo 105: Working the arms is probably the most difficult body part for students and new massage therapists to work on. Initially, there doesn't seem to be a whole lot of area to work on (yet working this area seems to help profoundly). During a Rolfing® session, I will use knuckles or fingers to do precise work on the arms. I have learned to love working on arms and get a kick out of the benefits to the shoulder that working on the biceps can bring! In this photo I am leaning forward to working on biceps brachii. Looking at this photo you may notice that I am not leaning from the ankles as much as I am leaning from my pelvis. This is because I don't need to exploit gravity as much in order work this particular area. If I needed more pressure, I would extend my hip a bit more and lean in more from my

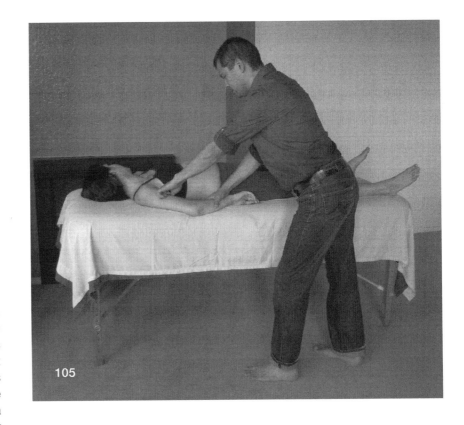

ankles. How do I come out of this stroke? Since I'm bending at my pelvis I usually bend my back knee slightly in order to bring my pelvis under my head then straighten out from there. Since I'm not bending over too much, the possible strain to my lower back is minimal. Integrate this stroke with non-deep-tissue massage and see how it works for you.

Photo 106: For a more blunt approach, I can use the same body mechanics but use a soft fist instead of knuckles. It's important to note that I am still leaning from my ankles but the lean doesn't need to be as much. As a side note, I

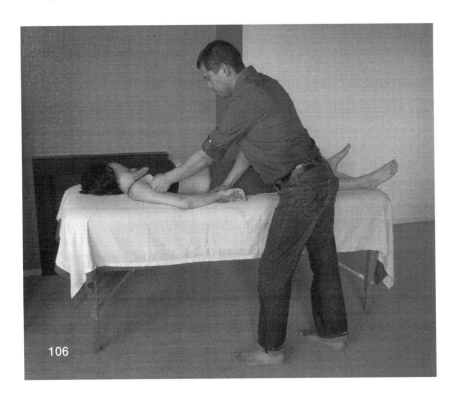

am holding my client's right hand. In this particular case, if I wasn't then her arm would move under my pressure. I would then have to conform and adapt my body to the abundant mobility of her arm. Since I need to target specific tissue in her arm, I am holding her arm down to do so. When using proper body mechanics, it's possible to exert a lot of pressure without much effort so care needs to be taken in the area I'm working on (the tendon of the long head of the biceps brachii is in this area). Be aware of your client's reactions when working any sensitive area and notice if they are entering FOF (pupils dilated, holding breath, tensing up, etc.). If so, back off until they are comfortable.

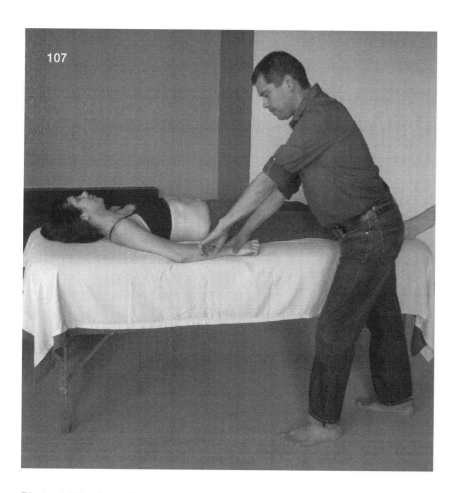

Photo 107: The most important thing to notice in this photo is the alignment of the bones of my left arm. My left palm is turned out. Doing so allows my radius and ulna to stack better on my humerus without muscular effort. If I were to leave my palm turned in, then my triceps and biceps need to tense up because my arm is more susceptible to flex under that position. When my palm is turned out (as in pronation), flexion of the elbow joint makes the least sense of any position. Instead, my metacarpals, carpals, radius, ulna, and humerus all stack to create one column that transfers the weight of my body onto the client's forearm. My shoulder stays relaxed and not raised. As I've mentioned before, if you are hyper flexible and this technique causes a hyperextension in the elbow joint, try another stroke that is safer for your body.

Photo 108: Sometimes working an area that you've always worked the same way can create a rut for you and the client. Changing things up occasionally can help to add variety to a session, spark a different way of thinking for the bodyworker, and help differentiate you from 'the crowd'. Instead of working the hand while standing and squeezing the fingers with your hands or driving thumbs into someone's thenar eminence, I like to half-sit on the table and bring the client's arm back, exposing the palm. Keeping my arms straight (but not locked) my straight fingers can work all the nooks and crannies of the hand (including the thenar eminence). I can only get force from my upper body as I'm sitting on the table so in this case I make the effort to be as specific as possible. If I felt any undue twisting in my body, I would counter that by putting more of my right leg on the table, keeping an appropriate distance from the client.

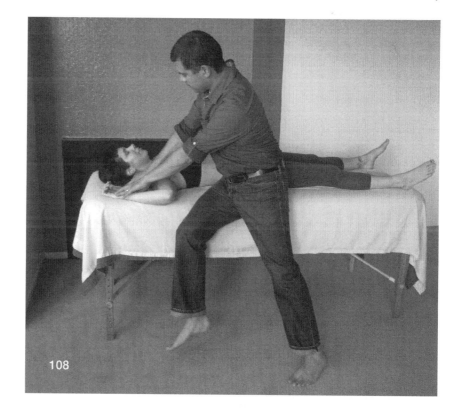

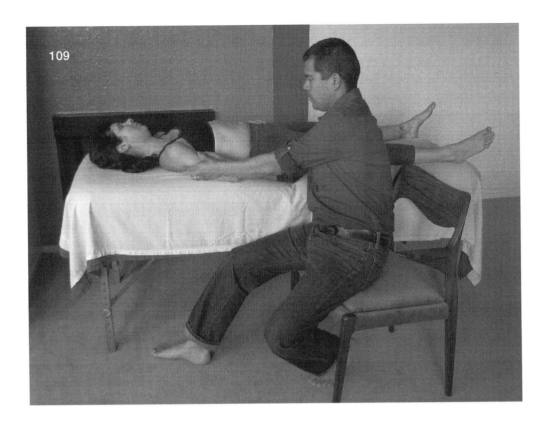

Photo 109: In Brazil I learned this method for working the triceps. A little bit of effort is necessary for the grip but the rest of the work is done by me leaning back and pulling on the tricep tissue. I sit on the edge of the chair in order to have enough space to lean back. Because I am working on specific tissue, I don't have to grip as much here but some gripping is necessary. Notice that even though I'm sitting, I still keep myself stable by keeping one foot forward. I am still in a forward stance of sorts.

Photo 110: A unique approach to working deeply on the forearms is this technique. Here I am getting some extra height by going up on my toes for a bit. I won't be on my toes for too long so doing so doesn't cause any undue strain. The middle knuckle of my soft fist travels along the interosseus membrane of the client's forearm. In this position, the forearm bones are very parallel and very open to the work. My right hand is on the client's right hand, which is on her ribcage. I am doing this in order to make sure my weight is going straight down and not into the client's ribcage. I make sure my shoulder is not raised and I'm keeping my arm close to my body in order to prevent any muscling in the shoulder girdle. I am mindful not to drop my head too much. This technique and way of using my body creates a tremendous amount of pressure on the forearm and can be reserved for very dense/muscular clients.

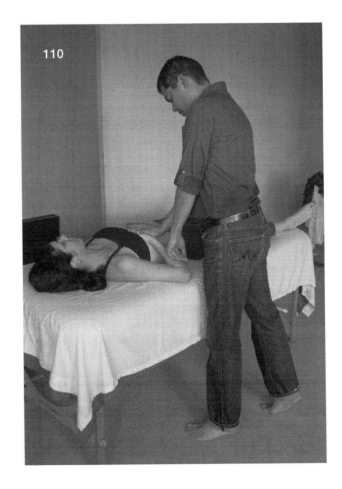

Working from the Midline

I have heard some students express to me the importance (as they have been told) of working from their midline and how some of my moves may not necessarily display that type of work. I understand the need to work from the midline but I also feel that it's more important to understand that the midline is a multiplanar line. Most practitioners will see the midline as a line running down the middle of their bodies and see it as a line that only goes in the forward and backward direction (along the sagittal plane). In fact, the midline can move either along the sagittal plane or the frontal plane or any other plane you can imagine. If we see it that way, then we can see ourselves tapping into a power and strength that has been the basis of the techniques I have shown. When students observe my work and ask me why I'm not working from the midline, in my perception I am, just not always in the forward direction they they're accustomed to seeing.

CHAPTER 9:

BODY MECHANICS FOR SIDE LYING AND OTHER POSITIONS

Side lying position is a great way to change the way you work and in turn decrease the possibility of doing the same thing over and over again thus reducing the chance of a repetitive strain. It's also a way to change things up and add variety to how you work with your clients. My mentor has often told the story of two fantastic massage therapists. They both did great work. One of them would do the same thing with their clients. Over and over again, he would do the same routine and although he was extremely good, some clients got bored. One client in particular asked around and got a referral to another massage therapist. On the first visit, the other massage therapist put the client in side lying position. The client had never been placed in side lying position and was quickly impressed by the massage therapist. The story goes to show that variety can be a good thing when working with clients on a regular basis. Placing a client in side lying position can break the routine and change not only the way you see the client, but also the way the client interprets the work.

I am asked by my students how often I put my clients in side lying position and I would have to say, very often! As I've mentioned before, I'm not a large muscular guy and having to find the best way to work (which can include getting on the table and placing clients on their sides) gives me the opportunity to do the work I want to do.

Getting on the Table

In a lot of photos you have seen me get on the table while the client is also on. I see it as a way of getting the most out of my body but am always aware of not invading my client's space. Being open to working while on the table is a way of thinking out of the box. It can be effortless work and can be seen not only as exploiting gravity but also as exploiting the table. Use the table as a resource to be able to employ deeper work while still using proper body mechanics. I understand that a lot of massage therapists work in a spa setting and there may be particular rules for working on the table or getting on the table while client is on. In my experience when I have worked in spas I have used a prop like a chair or a bench to be able to have the advantage of added height or to create a lean. One of the most important things to be aware of when working on the table is to remember that intention is key when getting on the table. There may be liability reasons for not getting on the table at your place of work which is understandable. Intention communicates a lot and if I can work with the intention of meeting a particular goal I believe that it shows in the work and the client can also feel it.

Getting attached to your work

We all have barriers that will stop us from working differently even though we may sincerely want to. We get caught up in habitual patterns that keep us from trying something new. Either from an aspect of fear or ego, we hold ourselves back if we don't keep an open mind to working differently. This is a very normal part of being a practitioner and shouldn't be regarded as a weakness. It's normal for us to be attached to working in the way that we've always been working even if we know that there is a better way. As I mentioned earlier, one reason for attachment is fear. We are afraid of the unknown and of what it would be like to work differently even though we may be told by a trusted source that our current body mechanics may not be the safest way of working. It is very common to stick to an old habit because it's comfortable and known rather than to seek the unknown.

Ego also plays a big part in attachment. Some instructors believe that once the ego has been fed, the practitioner will not be open to adopting a different way of working since he or she may believe they are already doing a great job. I believe the ego is just a mask for the underlying true emotion which is fear. Even though there is a better way of working, there is an internal mechanism called fear that may come off as ego and create an attachment to habitual patterns that may not serve us. I sometimes see it in my workshops and take care with students caught in that pattern to help them take their bodywork to a new level.

I offer up the following photos in order to suggest a different way of working. Proper body mechanics can also involve thinking outside of the box and using your body in ways that may not have been previously thought.

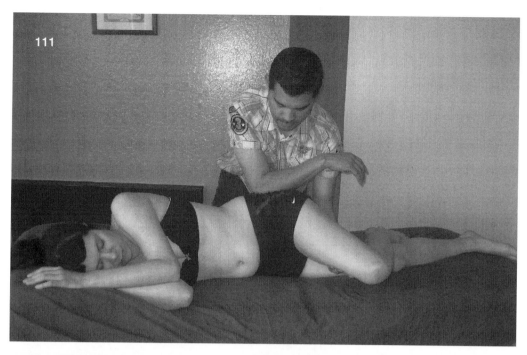

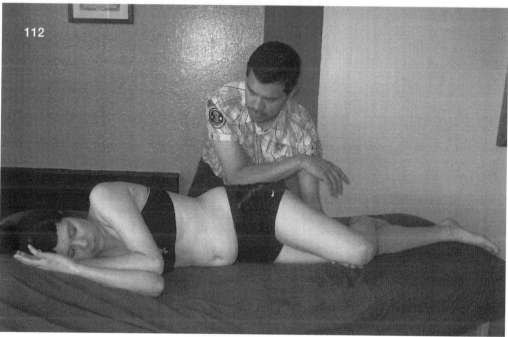

Photo 111 and Photo 112: In these photos my client is in side lying position and my right elbow and part of my ulna are working on an area right off her greater trochanter. If you can notice in the photo my right knee is on the table slightly. I am doing this to adjust to the height of the table. If I had an electric table, then I would just lower it but in this case I don't. When I can get a little more height then I can employ a little more pressure on the client's pelvis without effort. I'm not putting direct downward pressure on her pelvis so that I'm scrunching her pelvic bone together, instead the pressure goes down but slightly towards me so that I can work in line with the lateral rotators around the greater trochanter. Notice my right shoulder is slightly up. This is not an indication of muscular tension but instead it's because of what my left hand is doing. In photo 112 you can see that I am using my left hand to lift up the client's left leg. This shortens the lateral rotators and allows me to sink further into the tissue without 'muscling' it. This move also bring my left shoulder down making it look like my right shoulder is raised.

Photo 113: Another way of employing proper body mechanics and using gravity when working in side lying position is to have both knees on the table and use a soft fist instead of a forearm. Be aware of not getting too close to the client. My right soft fist is in the same area as before while my left hand is helping me to stabilize by resting on the IT band area. With both knees on the table I am off balance in the forward-backward direction and my left hand is helping to keep me balanced. If I want more pressure, I can lighten up on the left hand and make sure I'm off balance in the forward

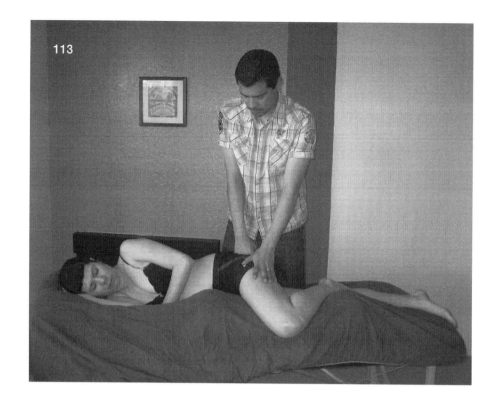

direction to apply more force (gravity) on the area. Be mindful to keep your wrists straight and all bones stacked. This is a great way to work muscle tissue that's not easily accessible in prone position and it's out of the box thinking when working the pelvis.

Photo 114: A variation is to use the same exact technique but instead of working on the lateral rotators I am now working on the quadratus lumborum. Looking and working with the body differently is a key ingredient to finding

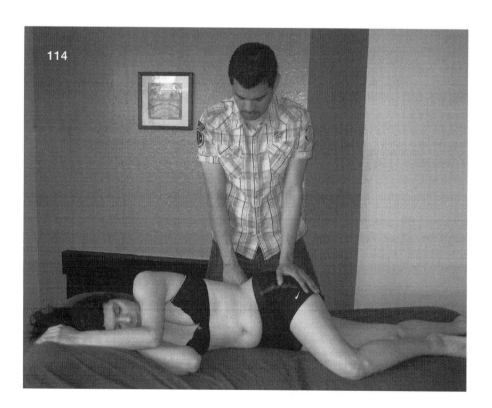

more efficient, effective, and safe ways to work. The knuckles of my soft fist are the ones working the area, with the intention of working the fascia between erectors and quadratus lumborum. This technique is not employing as much pressure as the previous techniques but I still need to ensure all bones are stacked and I'm not muscling it in order to avoid any undue strain. Notice I keep my arm close to my body. This is done in order to prevent strain in the shoulder girdle that can come about from having to stabilize an arm that's distant from the torso.

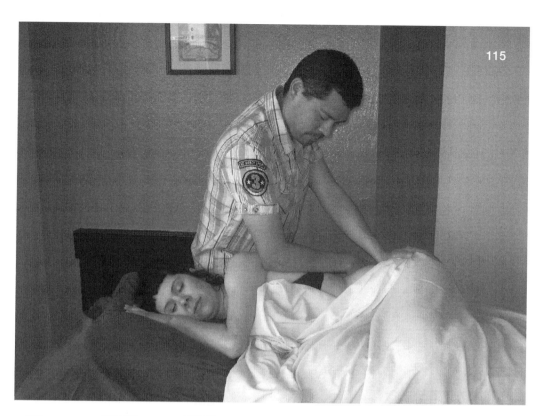

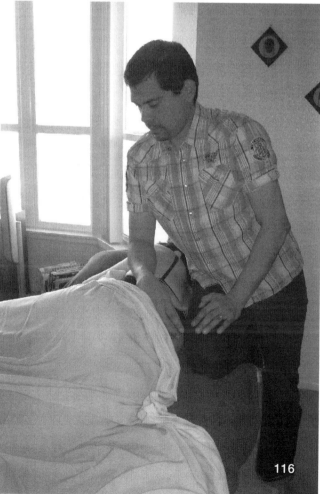

Photo 115 and Photo 116: In Photo 115, instead of using a soft fist or knuckles to work on my clients teres muscle group, I am halfway kneeling on the table and leaning into the teres muscle groups with my forearm. My torso is not flexed and my forearm is close to my torso to avoid strain. I'm about to ask the client to move her left arm out towards your head so that the muscle tissue is stretched under my forearm, making my work more effective without any additional effort. The next photo shows how my leg is on the table. It's important to note that I am not raising the table height up or down and instead I am adapting to the table height itself. If you're working in a spa and the table height was fixed or you didn't have time to change the table height (remember, back to back to back clients) this is an alternative. This is just one of many examples that shows there are ways to work around table height and for our bodies to adapt to table height in order to make for effective work. In photo 116 I moved my left hand to my right knee to show how my right wrist is relaxed.

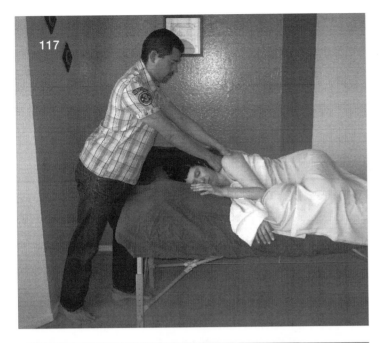

Photo 117: Working in sideline position allows me to work the upper trapezius muscle from a different angle. I purposefully placed the table closer to a wall in order to show that this technique is great when working in a smaller space. A lot of massage therapists have little space to work with and this is a great way to work the upper trapezius area and supraspinatus with minimal effort. Notice it doesn't seem as if I'm leaning in much but I am able to produce deep tissue work with a small amount of lean from my ankles. My soft fist goes downward in this move in order to exploit gravity, I do not work upward. This is only possible if I employ my ankles and keep my arm relatively straight. My other hand is on my client's shoulder in order to stabilize it.

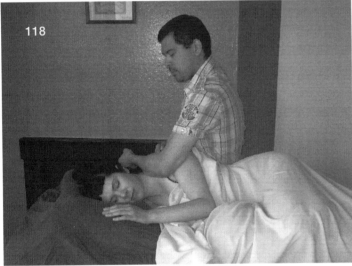

Photo 118: In this photo I am still working the upper trapezius muscle using the ulna part of my forearm but now I am sitting with part of my left leg on the table behind the client and my right-hand stabilizing the clients shoulder while my left forearm is scooping out the upper part of the trapezius. My whole body is doing the movement as I lean back and scoop at the same time instead of having to muscle it. This produces great deep work that isn't too pointy. I make sure to not be flexed and not to let my head drop.

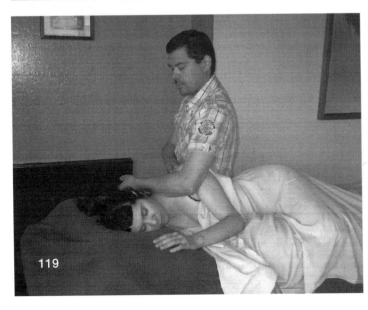

Photo 119: Here I show another angle of the same technique showing my arm first scoops then supinates in order to work the tissue. My arm isn't moving medial to lateral on the upper trapezius as that would make me raise my shoulder and create a pattern for strain. Any lateral movement comes out as a result of my also leaning back and taking my forearm in the same direction of the lean. A note on draping and putting someone in side lying position while they are draped: Back in school we were taught to use 3 to 4 pillows when propping a client in side lying position. If you want to put someone in side lying position just for a few minutes to work a particular part of the body don't feel it's necessary to make it a big production to do so. I have one pillow that I put underneath the client's head and I used the bolster that was under her feet to put under her top leg. It took less than half a minute to do this and from this point I can put the client back into either prone or supine position fairly easily.

Photo 120: This photo shows how simple it is to work the neck in sideline position. Notice I am working with my fingers. My knuckles and wrists are straight as well as my arm and because of this all the energy can flow through my arm (energy in this case is the force of gravity) I am leaning forward and can easily and effortlessly place pressure on to the client's neck, pressure that is coming from me leaning forward. My right knee is on the table and I am doing this because the table height has been effectively raised by having the client in sideline position. The client's neck receives as much of my upper body weight as I choose to place.

Specificity is key also as my fingers are in the posterior triangle area (behind sternocleidomastoid and in front of the trapezius) which doesn't require a lot of pressure. Since my right leg is bent at the knee and is on the table I have to flex my hip flex to lean forward and use my upper body weight to work on the client's neck.

Photo 121: Thinking outside the box is important when adapting to a person on the table and adapting to how your body is moving or is not moving. In photo 121 I go down on one knee and work the clients forearm. Notice my thumb is in the area of the interosseous membrane. I am actually not grasping with my thumb but my thumb is actually maintaining one point along the client's forearm as my right hand is helping the forearm go into supination. I may do this technique if I have limited work space or if I don't have a stool or chair. I encourage you to use this book as a catalyst for finding different ways of working with your clients.

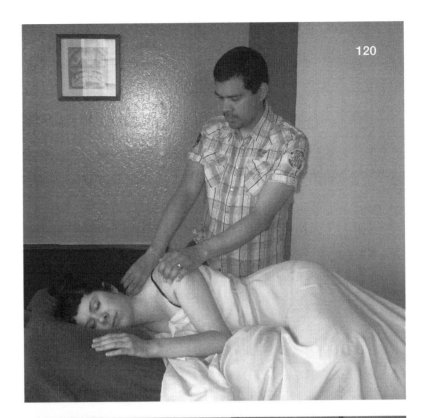

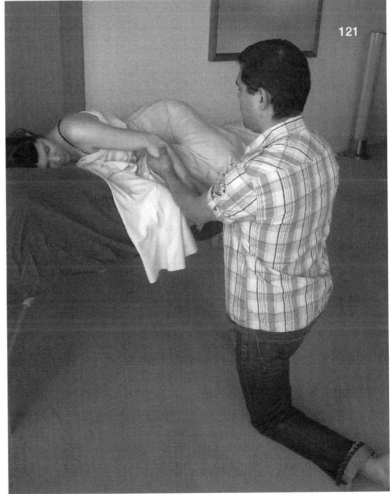

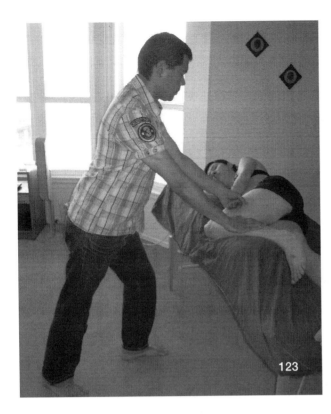

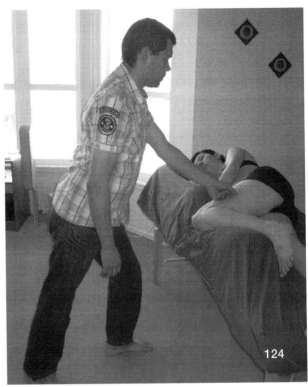

Photos 123 and 124: In working the IT band in side lying position I am using the soft fist as the tool however my whole body is involved in this technique. All the bones of my arm are in line properly so that when I lean forward it takes a minimal amount of leaning in order to get the job done. As you can tell it seems almost as if I'm standing up but I actually just have to lean slightly in order to sink deeper into the tissue. The photo shows how much leaning is necessary and how relaxed the practitioner can be in doing deep work. In photo 123 my right hand is still holding the client's leg for support. No actual weight is being placed on that hand. Photo 124 shows the right hand down in order to see the left arm fully. Notice the arm is aligned, my ankles are being employed, and my whole body is relatively straight, as if in the vertical version of the plank pose in yoga. Similar to plank pose, my transversus abdominis muscles are engaged but not overly contracted. As with other techniques that use soft fist, I will travel along the IT band only up to the point that my wrist is still straight and aligned with my forearm muscles. Once my wrist starts to bend or twist, I ease up and try a different technique. Finally, my left arm and left leg are forward, reminding us of a boxer's jab.

Photos 125: In this photo I am using a forearm instead of a soft fist to work on the IT band. Notice I can create a lot of pressure by leaning from the ankle joints and also slightly leaning from the pelvis. My left hand is relaxed my head is not dropped and although it may seem as if there is compression on my right hand I'm not actually putting any pressure on my right hand just stabilizing myself. It doesn't take a whole lot of leaning to get deep into this tissue when working in side lying position. How long would I be in this position? I actually won't be here very long once I sink into the tissue but what may take some time is slowly allowing more of my gravity to create pressure on the client's IT band. Because of this I may be holding back from leaning too much on my client. I would use my front leg to take on my upper body weight until I can sink deeper into the IT band. Of course, this will require focus and paying attention to what the tissue is telling you.

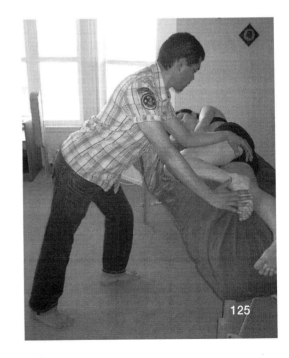

Photo 126: Working from across the table can have its advantages and disadvantages. If the table height is too high then I may not be able to get the proper access to tissue. If the table height is too low then I may actually be incurring back strain by leaning over across the table. In this photo I am leaning over across the table to work on the client's abductor and lower leg region. Although I'm leaning forward I am not putting strain on my low back. This is because my arms are essentially supporting me while also working on the client's abductor and lower leg region. I also keep the forward stance and that helps a lot, allowing me to stand up easily by using my front leg and not using my lower back muscles. This work is more of a compression technique and less of a stroke so I'm moving up and down the leg with slow steady compressions, as I shift my body up and down the leg.

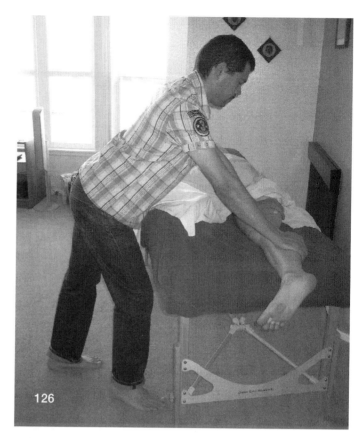

126

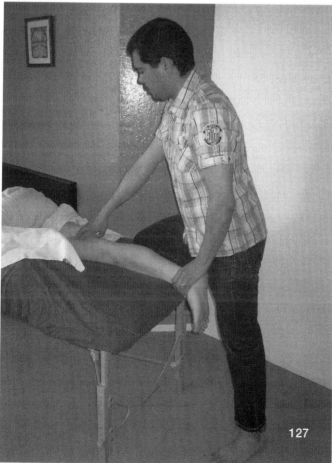

127

Photo 127: This photo shows a different way of working, here my knuckles are 'parked' along the abductors. My left hand is holding the leg and has it internally rotated. My right knee is on the table to allow me to get additional height in order to have my right arm come down more on the adductor tissue. When working this way I imagine my whole body is in a yoga plank position and leaning forward with the exception of my right leg being on the table. This allows me to use very little of my upper body to create pressure on the client's adductors.

Photos 128 and 129: Slight detail work on the foot can be performed in sideline position as seen in these photos. My left knuckles are working in a small area of the medial arch of the right foot. My right hand is supporting the foot as I lean in with my left knuckles. I still have one foot forward and I'm still leaning into this area. In this case I deviated and placed my right foot forward although I am mainly working through my left hand. This shows how it is possible to change the technique but still keep the principle of exploiting gravity. If I want to apply more pressure I could lean into it more from my ankles but I've decided to show a different way that still exploits gravity. What I do in photo 129 is get more vertical so that more of my weight goes downward into the foot. Notice the heel of my left foot has come up and I am slightly on my toes. This allows me to gain more vertical downward pressure on to the client but my knuckles and my wrist are still in a straight line and my shoulder is not raised, I am still in a relaxed posture as I am working deeply into the client's foot.

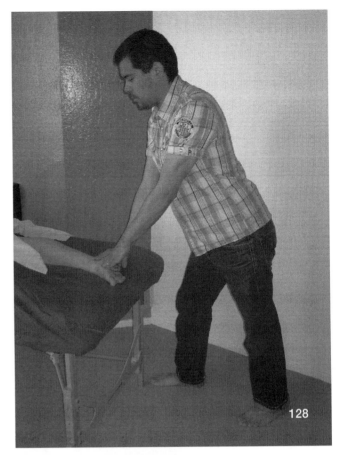

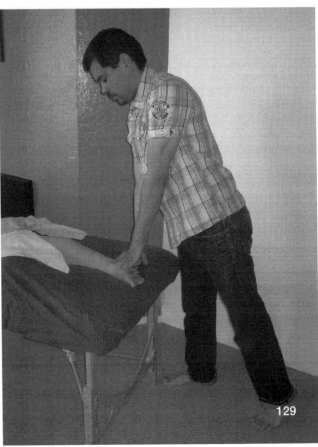

Photo 130: Here I'm exploring a way to give a stretch to the clients low back area, namely the quadratus lumborum, in side lying position. Once again my knee, in this case my right knee, is on the table which allows me to be off-balance in the direction of the clients head and my right hand is on her rib cage allowing me to anchor that area. My left hand is holding the client's left leg and I can bring a stretch to this area by bringing her left leg down off the table. Being in this off-balance position allows me to stretch and move her in different directions. For example, I can rotate towards my left and bring her left pelvis into further extension. Another thing I can do is keep the leg in a fixed position as I lean forward and bring myself further into off-balance but my right hand places more pressure on her serratus anterior tissue, working the fascia there.

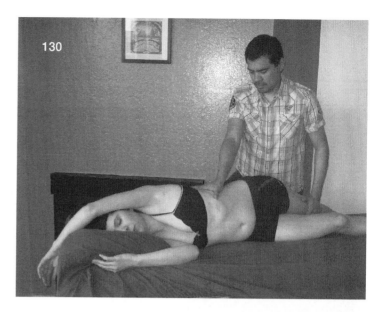

Photo 131: Here I am working the client's serratus anterior muscle. Both of my hands are straight in a forward position almost in a superman pose as I'm leaning forward into the tissue under the scapula. My toes are not curled and my feet are not completely splayed out. Keeping the toes and feet relaxed allows me to maintain further relaxation in my body and just leaning a little bit forward in this position let's me sink into the client's tissue efficiently and effectively and safely. In this manner my whole body is involved in the work and I am able to better feel what is happening under my hands. As some instructors call it, I am working with 'soft hands.'

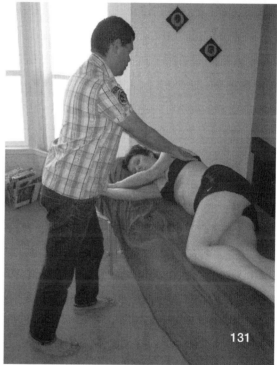

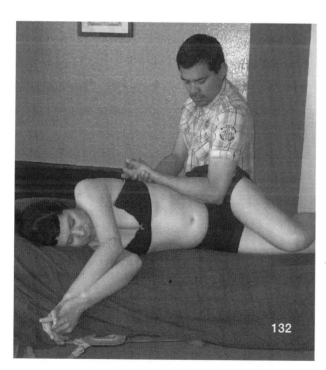

Photo 132: Working in side lying and using the table as a work aide allows you to work on muscle tissue in a different way than before. In this photo I am working the iliacus tissue in that area of the pelvis. With my left forearm I am sinking into that area of the pelvis and using my right hand to stabilize the left elbow. I'm sitting on the table and can lean back and use my body weight to further sink into that tissue. My left thigh is slightly on the table but I'm not completely sitting comfortably on the table, instead I'm a little off-balance. This off-balance allows me to exploit gravity in order to be able to lean back and sink into the iliacus tissue, via my body weight.

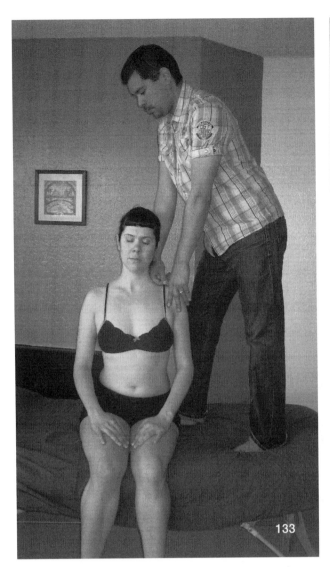
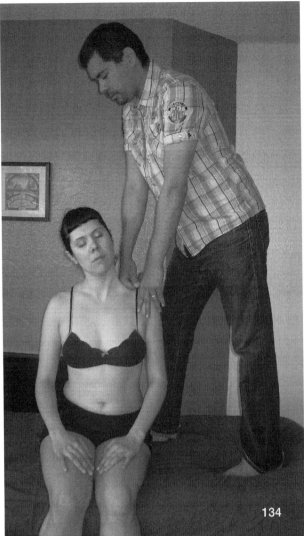

Photos 133 and 134: In these two photos I am standing on the table and my soft fist is working on the clients upper trapezius muscles. In this position I'm able to put a large percentage of my weight onto that muscle tissue since my soft fist and arm are lined up. Aligning the joints allows for easy transfer of my weight onto the client's muscle tissue. I only need to lean slightly in order to accomplish deep work. In photo 134 I am asking the client to slowly side-bend their neck which stretches the trapezius underneath my soft fist. This allows me to use even less muscle effort and just slowly lean into the muscle tissue as the client moves their head. I keep in my arm close to my body and make sure my shoulder girdle is not straining and that all pressure is going vertically into the muscle tissue. I have done this in the spa setting and save it for the end of the sessions. Let's say my client wanted focus on the shoulders. Once we're done I tell them to re-dress and let them know I will work on them for about a minute on their shoulder muscles in sitting position. If you do this with confidence then the client will be fine with it. You will be able to work differently than other massage therapist and this makes you stand out from the crowd in the client's mind. This out-of-the-box manner of working makes for a memorable session.

Photo 135: This is a move I love and learned at my training at the Rolf Institute. This technique clearly demonstrates a different approach to working the back. Here the client is on the table and I am on as well behind her using soft fists to work along the erector muscles. I still have one foot forward and my arms are still straight and although I am not in a plank pose or with my body straight my upper body is now being used to hinge forward and I'm still using gravity to have my upper body weight rest on the client's erectors via my soft fist. Again this is a different way of working and thinking, being able to work deeply with little effort.

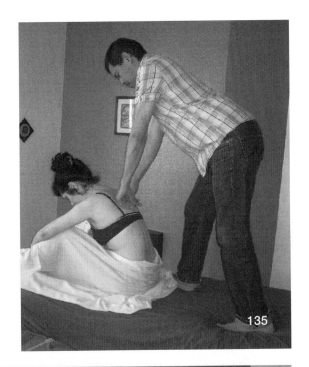

Photos 136 and 137: These photos show a modification of working the back. Here I have the client in a yoga pose called child's pose and I am leaning forward, my arms are straight and I'm able to work her lower back muscles by bending my knees in order to drop lower. I do not have a preference for either way of working but I do sometimes use knuckles instead of soft fist and I may sometimes lower my body just a bit in order to carry the proper angle of work lower, the closer I get to the client's pelvic bone. I find it very stimulating to find different ways of working and the client also appreciates the variety when I put them in different positions. Another thing that I find very interesting about working this way is that it's almost more difficult to muscle it when employing proper body mechanics. My wrists and arms are straight but not locked and my back is not overly curved and not flat, just a normal curve. I am hinging from my pelvis and easily work the client's lumbar fascia. Photo 137 shows how I can move my left leg back if I wanted to keep it straight. In order to stand up from this position I would bend my left leg in order to bring my pelvis under my head then stand up from there.

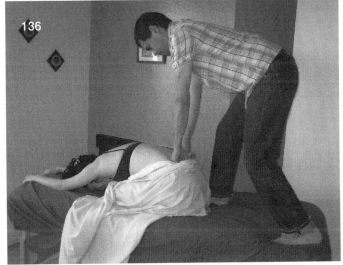

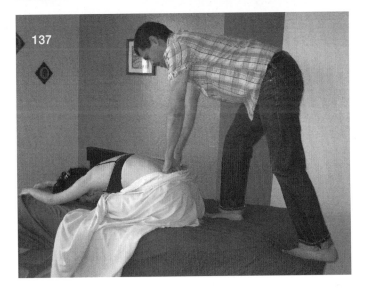

Proper body mechanics can lead to an injury free and successful practice. Not only are you working with less strain, but you will be less tired when working on clients, possibly being able to see one more client in a month than before. Using your imagination to work outside the box yet still use proper body mechanics will make you stand out from the crowd and differentiate you in the client's mind. Using your body properly will also keep you fit since you will be using your whole body to do your work and not just your upper or lower body. I personally attribute proper body mechanics to a lot of positive aspects of my practice and because of this I wish to share this knowledge with you. I hope the information in this book helps you as it has helped me. If the contents of this book inspires you to do one thing differently in your practice and in turn remove even a bit of strain from your body, then it would have been well worth reading. Enjoy mastering body mechanics!

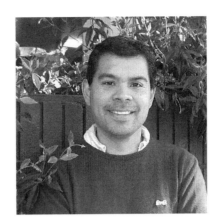

ABOUT THE AUTHOR

Marty Morales is a Certified Rolfer™ and Rolf Movement Practitioner™. Having taken up Reflexology in 1996 to help his wife manage Crohn's Disease, Marty eventually turned his hobby into a career by pursuing massage therapy training in 2002. Over the years, Marty has had extensive experience working at high-end spas, chiropractic offices, and at sporting events.

Eventually, the passion for bodywork evolved into the desire for sharing that passion and in 2005, Marty started teaching at the San Francisco School of Massage. Marty has taught beginning and advanced level classes and has held numerous advanced bodywork workshops in subjects ranging from Deep Tissue Massage to Medical Massage. Marty also travels to spas to provide body mechanics consulting. An interest in body movement and awareness (through studies of Judo and Jiu Jitsu) led to pursuing Rolfing® and Rolf Movement training in Brazil in 2008.

In addition to doing and teaching bodywork, Marty blends his current and previous knowledge (MBA in Finance) to provide business coaching and marketing classes to massage therapists.

Marty lives in San Francisco with his wife Elena, and maintains a thriving practice while teaching throughout Northern California.

Made in the USA
San Bernardino, CA
12 August 2014